**Dr. Alan H. Pressman D.C., Ph.D., D.A.C.B.N., C.C.N.,** is a chiropractor and a board certified dietitian/nutritionist. He is the former chairman of the Department of Clinical Nutrition at New York Chiropractic College and served numerous terms as president for the Council on Nutrition of the American Chiropractic Association. He is also a diplomate and past president of the American Chiropractic Board of Nutrition.

Dr. Pressman has been a regular contributor on CNBC, and is a noted veteran radio guest on ABC and WOR talk radio. His expertise on a wide range of topical health issues has been heard by millions on the nationally syndicated radio show, *Dr. Pressman on Health* on WEVD (10.50 AM-NY). He is currently the director of Gramercy Health Associates in New York City.

**Herbert D. Goodman, M.D., Ph.D., F.A.D.E.P.,** is a noted medical practitioner of both traditional and alternative medicine. His specialties include emergency medicine, pain management, acupuncture, geriatrics, and hypnosis.

Dr. Goodman is a Fellow in the American Academy of Disability Evaluating Physicians, a diplomate in the American Academy of Pain Management, and was elected as an approved consultant for the American Society of Clinical Hypnosis. He is currently director of the Southwestern Center for Pain in Phoenix, Arizona.

D0837315

# THE PHYSICIANS' GUIDES TO HEALING

---

# TREATING ARTHRITIS, CARPAL TUNNEL SYNDROME, AND JOINT CONDITIONS

*Alan Pressman, D.C., Ph.D., D.A.C.B.N., C.C.N.,
and Herbert D. Goodman, M.D., Ph.D.,
with Karen Lane*

*Developed by The Philip Lief Group, Inc.*

**IB**

**BERKLEY BOOKS, NEW YORK**

TREATING ARTHRITIS, CARPAL TUNNEL SYNDROME, AND
JOINT CONDITIONS

A Berkley Book / published by arrangement with
The Philip Lief Group, Inc.

PRINTING HISTORY
Berkley edition / May 1997

The Putnam Berkley World Wide Web site address is
http://www.berkley.com

ISBN: 0-425-15694-X

BERKLEY®
Berkley Books are published by The Berkley Publishing Group,
200 Madison Avenue, New York, New York 10016.
BERKLEY and the "B" design
are trademarks belonging to Berkley Publishing Corporation.

PRINTED IN THE UNITED STATES OF AMERICA

10  9  8  7  6  5  4  3  2  1

# THE PHYSICIANS' GUIDES TO HEALING

---

## TREATING ARTHRITIS, CARPAL TUNNEL SYNDROME, AND JOINT CONDITIONS

# Contents

# Introduction

## ARE YOU HEALTHY?

The answer to the above question may depend upon whom you ask. Allopathic medicine, also called conventional, traditional, or Western medicine, defines health as the absence of disease. In the allopathic tradition, chemical medications and surgical operations are the primary tools of healing. Much of the power to heal relies upon the progress of modern technology for its theories and practices. By contrast, holistic—also called alternative or natural medicine—is based on preventive care and focuses not only bodily health but on psychological and spiritual health as well. To the holistic practitioner, good health is as much a reflection of our lifestyle and emotional stability as it is a product of avoiding disease and eating the proper foods. In the holistic vision of wellness, a balanced union of physical, spiritual, and emotional states produces vibrancy and longevity.

Clearly, allopathic and holistic practitioners approach health care from different vantage points. But there has been a revolution within the traditional medical establishment and a new era has begun—one that integrates alternative therapy and theories of overall wellness with allopathic medicine and rigorous practices of surgery and pharmaceuticals. Also known as complementary medicine, the fusion of the two schools of medicine has become the new frontier of health care. At last, patients can benefit from the collective wisdom of both ideologies of medical thought.

The *Physicians' Guides to Healing* series has been developed to give readers insight into the benefits of complementary medicine on a variety of health issues. The series consists of five authoritative health reference books, each of which provides accurate and up-to-date information on treatments from the perspectives of allopathic, alternative, and complementary medicine. The titles in the series—*Treating Asthma, Allergies, and Food Sensitivities; Treating Arthritis, Carpal Tunnel Syndrome, and Joint Conditions; Treating Hypertension and Other Cardiovascular Diseases; Treating Gynecological Conditions;* and *Treating Digestive Conditions*—will help the reader understand and compare both allopathic and alternative approaches to specific health problems, and make informed decisions about which combination of therapies is best suited to individual needs.

Dr. Herbert Goodman and Dr. Alan Pressman, coauthors of the series, lend their unsurpassed medical expertise to each volume. Both practitioners incorporate elements of natural medicine into their own traditional practices, approaching their patients' needs in a broad-minded and sensitive manner. Each book in the series reflects their confidence in complementary medicine and includes several case studies that closely examine the health problems and genuine concern of real people. These case histories demonstrate the potential healing power of complementary therapy when all else has failed, and they show how a candid and trusting relationship between doctor and patient is essential to effective and precise treatment.

Although the goals of both allopathic and alternative medicine are similar—health, immunity to diseases, and well-being—the approaches of holistic care focus more on preparing the body for a lifetime of total body health through healthy living, natural healing, and overall wellness rather than on curing specific illnesses as they arise. The various areas of alternative medicine include: mind/body control, as displayed in studies of art, dance, music therapy, biofeedback, yoga, and psychotherapy; manual healing therapies, such as acupressure, Alexander technique, chiropractic, massage, osteopathy, reflexology, and therapeutic touch; bioelectromagnetic therapy involving techniques such as blue light, artificial lighting, electrostimulation, and neuromagnetic stimulation; diet and nutrition, including vitamins, nutritional supplements, and practices like Gerson therapy; and herbal medicine, among other options. These are a few of the holistic remedies that you will become familiar with as you read the *Physicians' Guides to Healing*.

Of course, traditional treatments offer just as wide a range of possibilities and countless benefits. For instance, without the technology of modern surgical procedures and the mechanics of pacemakers, many people who suffer from irregular heartbeats would not be able to survive; likewise, without specialists' knowledge of orthopedic reconstruction operations, torn ligaments and deteriorated cartilage would prevent many injured people from walking. Cancerous tumors, including breast cancer, might claim the lives of thousands of cancer patients were it not for allopathic procedures such as mastectomies. Millions of cancer patients have extended their lives and improved their chances of survival with treatments such as surgery, radiation, and chemotherapy.

# TRADITIONAL MEDICINE: A BRIEF HISTORY

Our knowledge of traditional medicine dates back as far as written history, although prescientific healing practices were based on magic, talismans, spells, incantations, and folk remedies ("old wives' tales"). Rudimentary surgery from the days before scientific medicine involved procedures such as trepanning, which entailed boring holes in the skull to relieve headaches, insanity, and epilepsy. As early as the third century B.C. doctors gained status as scientists, distinct from sorcerers and priests. Egyptian doctors are reported to have been trained for their profession by learning the arts of interrogation, inspection, and palpation (examination by touch). The drugs available to the Egyptians, though primitive, are still in use today, including figs, dates, and castor oil for laxatives purposes; and tannic acid to soothe and treat burns. Early Mesopotamians also discovered a wealth of primitive pharmaceuticals in various forms, many of which were derived from mineral sources. The Mesopotamians are renowned for being the first society to develop accurate models of the liver, which they regard as "the seat of the soul." This was the dawn of pharmacology, anatomy, and physiology.

The teachings of Hippocrates, the "father of medicine" who lived in Greece during the third century B.C., are the foundation of the modern medical values. His Hippocratic oath, which established a code of medical honor, is a vow of integrity that people in the health care industry take even today. Herophilus, an Egyptian from the same time period, is reported to have performed the first public dissection of a human cadaver. The founder of comparative anatomy was the Greek philosopher Aristotle, who also publicly performed dissections of many animals. According to etched records, early Egyptians performed castrations, removal of bladder stones, amputations, and various optical surgeries. Hindus in the second and third centuries A.D. performed the first known plastic surgery by grafting skin from the thigh and buttocks onto the nose. Chinese drugs in the same period included rhubarb, aconite, sulfur, animal organs, and—most importantly—opium, a powerful and effective pain reliever and anesthetic. The interest in the human body, the study of various types of life forms, and these early attempts at surgery and remedial drug use provided the foundations for the rest of medical evolution.

The Middle Ages in Europe were times of scientific advances as more empirical and physical knowledge accumulated among learned men. The Italians were the first people to officially separate science from religion in the ninth and tenth centuries, allowing progress to be propelled by research and analysis—not faith. In the thirteenth century, several countries including France and Italy saw the formation of the medieval guilds, which were social class rankings based upon profession. Barbers had always performed elementary surgery until the establishment of guilds. At that point, surgeons gained increased training, respect, and social status while barbers resigned themselves to haircutting and beard-shaving. In 1543, the publication of a treatise called *On the Structure of the Human Body* by the Belgian anatomist Andreas Vesalius prompted a surge in medical research and the development of new physiological discoveries. In the same decade, colleagues and students of Vesalius made the first diagnoses of ear diseases and the identification of fallopian tubes, eye muscles, tear ducts, and they arrived at the notion of a circulatory system.

The most important milestone in seventeenth-century medicine was the discovery by English physician William

Harvey, of the exact mechanism of blood circulation, a discovery that incited closer studies of the heart, lungs, and lymph systems as well. The introduction of quinine—a drug used to treat tuberculosis patients—was a major event in therapeutic progress during the seventeenth century. During this same period, French physician Ambroise Paré was nicknamed "the father of modern surgery" because he discovered that ligating arteries with a red-hot iron could be used to control bleeding and increase the patient's chances for survival. This discovery enabled doctors to perform surgery without worrying about time constraints or their patient's death from blood loss.

The notion of germs was taken quite seriously by nineteenth-century medical practitioners, and the use of carbolic acid (believed to kill germs) became a reliable way to reduce the likelihood of wound infections. Contributions to the understanding of shock management and antibiotic administration also greatly increased success rates in surgery. Other contributions from this century include X rays, discovered accidentally by Dr. Wilhelm Conrad Röntgen in Germany, and the use of ultraviolet radiation for treating many skin diseases, including psoriasis and tuberculosis of the skin. American scientists contributed significant research and understanding to operative gynecology: in 1809, Ephraim McDowell of Kentucky performed the first successful removal of an ovarian tumor, marking the dawn of modern surgical procedure in the United States. Although medicine was rapidly achieving new and amazing goals, there were inevitable failures. For example, in the eighteenth century, John Brown promoted the theory that disease was caused by a lack of stimulation, and he therefore proposed stimulating his patients into health by bombarding them with "heroic" doses of poisonous drugs like mercuric chloride. Needless to say, not all of Dr. Brown's remedies resulted in restoring vigor and health to his patients.

The development of new ideas and technologies in the twentieth century has exponentially increased the magnitude of physical, chemical, surgical, and pharmacological knowledge. In addition to contributing to a general improvement in living conditions and a greater awareness of health issues, science has progressed into the realms of the previously inconceivable and impossible. For example, in the field of genetics, DNA replication is now possible; ultrasound technology makes viewing the fetus a normal prenatal procedure; and human life is readily created outside the woman's body by means of *in vitro* fertilization. And who would have believed that body parts could be reattached to the body, enabling dead tissue to come back to life? In 1962, the first successful limb replacement was performed: an arm, completely severed at the shoulder, was rejoined. Synthetic materials now allow surgeons to perform surgical replacements of hips, arms, teeth, and so on. Additionally, kidney and other organ transplants are now routinely successful.

Infectious diseases are largely under control now that most people have access to improved antibiotics, vaccines, and sanitation. The "wonder drugs" of the nineteenth and twentieth centuries have virtually wiped out most major diseases: sulfonamide antibiotics treat syphilis; streptomycin kills tuberculosis; sulfones treat leprosy; quinine treats malaria. Vaccines were developed for almost all of the most threatening epidemic diseases; for smallpox (1796), typhoid fever (1897), diphtheria (1923), tetanus (1930s) and for yellow fever, measles, mumps, and rubella. The discovery of penicillin in 1938 by Englishmen Howard Florey and Ernst Chain vastly reduced World War II fatalities and continues to effectively treat many types of infections. Genetic engineering, a concept that originated in the 1980s, led to the development of vaccines for herpes simplex, hepatitis B, influenza, and chicken pox. In general, scientists and physicians now have a vastly improved understanding of the human body's immune system and can therefore anticipate and eliminate most significant health hazards. Even with modern-day health horrors such as AIDS, the Ebola virus, and increased cancer incidence rates, we can have faith that science will eventually find more and better treatments for such diseases.

Cardiovascular disease, one of the most threatening contemporary medical conditions, has recently become less of an enigma thanks to imaging techniques like magnetic resonating imagery (MRI) developed in the 1970s. Cardiac catheterization, which enables measurements of pressure to be taken in the heart, helps doctors analyze potential heart conditions. Also, an array of drugs—including chemicals that have been developed to block certain functions of the sympathetic nervous system—is now available to treat angina, heart arrhythmia, and hypertension. Bypass surgery (replacing arteries damaged or narrowed by cholesterol buildup) and the transplantation of temporary and permanent artificial hearts have greatly widened options for sufferers of cardiovascular conditions. Such inventions and discoveries, complemented with essential nutritional information on reducing cholesterol, sodium, and fat intake, make controlling cardiovascular risk factors easier.

The new horizons in modern medicine promise a wealth of possibilities. Some practices that are now in their incipient stages with great promises for the future include cryogenics (freezing blood in surgeries such as those for Parkinson's disease and for brain tumors), psychopharmacology (which has virtually replaced the barbaric practice of prefrontal lobotomy), microsurgery (used, for example, to operate on the inner ear), the use of plastics (silicon and Teflon) to replace defective body parts, and transplantation (of teeth, liver, hearts, endocrine glands).

Modern medicine has evolved considerably since the days of trepanning, bloodletting with leeches, and induced purgation with mercuric chloride. Allopathic practitioners have begun to incorporate holistic therapies into their treatment programs, and they have accepted many of the ideas that were once only acknowledged by alternative practitioners, some of which are described below. The result: a progressive, preventive approach to healing, and the widely accepted conviction that complementary medicine works wonders. In 1992 the federal government established the Office of Alternative Medicine as part of the National Institutes of Health (NIH)—conclusive proof that alternative medicine has indeed entered the mainstream.

## ALTERNATIVE MEDICINE: A BRIEF HISTORY

Natural medicine has always existed in various manifestations. Even before the advent of technological innovations and chemical research, human beings have taken the steps necessary to restore good health by using any remedy that appeared to positively affect their ailments. Long before modern pain medicine, Native Americans chewed on willow bark to relieve pain and headaches. Nowadays people are more likely to reach for a couple of aspirin tablets, but the principle is the same: willow contains salicylic acid, the same ingredient used to produce aspirin. We all want to drink ginger ale when we're feeling sick, but do you know the reason why? The properties of the herbal ginger root are known to settle stomachaches. Even if carbonated ginger ale hasn't been around for centuries, ginger tonic certainly has. The principles of natural healing have inspired many noninvasive cures for pain and illness throughout history. Throughout history Eastern medicine has been particularly successful in finding natural cures and using the body's inherent ability to heal itself from within. Much of what we consider "alternative" is simply Eastern in origin.

One of the oldest recorded alternative treatments is acupuncture, which dates back to 2000 B.C. Chinese healers developed acupuncture in response to the theory that there are special points known as meridians on the body connected to the internal organs and that vital energy flows along the lines that connect the meridians. According to this theory, diseases are caused by interruptions in the energy flow; inserting and twirling acupuncture needles into certain meridian points can stimulate energy and restore the body's normal energy flow. Acupuncture is widely used today in most Chinese hospitals for relieving pain, but only about ten percent of American practitioners have recognized its efficacy and use it to treat patients. It is used as an analgesic for a wide variety of problems and is commonly employed in the treatment of brain surgery, ulcers, hypertension, asthma, and various heart conditions. The modern, physiological explanation for why and how acupuncture works, according to American neurophysiologists, is based on the theory that endorphins and enkephalins (the body's natural painkillers) are released when the skin is pierced by needles.

In the late eighteenth century, in defiance of the common medical procedure resulting from theories such as Dr. Brown's, Samuel Hahneman devised a theory that "likes are cured by likes," meaning that the body's natural defenses could be implemented to cure any ailment with the help of natural, botanical stimulants. Hahneman's theory was the birth of homeopathy as we know it today. His idea of using the elements already available to us in nature (such as chamomile flowers or Kombucha mushrooms) and within our own bodies (such as our highly complex and effective immune system) gave birth to a set of practices that continues to generate innovative techniques for holistic healing today. Homeopathy was introduced to the United States in 1825, and the American Institute of Homeopathy was founded in 1844.

An important milestone in the development of holistic medicine was the emergence of naturopathy, which means "natural curing." In 1902 a German doctor named Benedict Lust brought his theory of naturopathy to America. He had been impressed by the benefits he had witnessed in Europe when people who visited water spas would return refreshed, relaxed, and invigorated. He recognized that nature's abundant natural resources—like water and sun—could be tapped and utilized as great healing agents. Water curing has always been an effective therapeutic treatment; just think of relaxing in a hot tub or taking a long hot shower to unwind after a stressful day of work. The term *hydrotherapy* was coined shortly after Hahneman imported the idea to America. In some European countries today, a visit to the health spa for a water cure is covered by health insurance. Dr. Lust is responsible for a wider acceptance of natural medicine during his time than in any other period in modern medicine, present day excluded. He also believed in preventive measures such as good diet, exercise, mud baths, chiropractic massage, and other natural treatments. These fundamental tenets, along with Samuel Hahneman's, are still the cornerstones of holistic medicine today.

The major advancement of health care technology, especially in areas of surgery and pharmacology in the 1930s, is responsible for some of the deep segregation between homeopathic and traditional medicine. Earlier this century, there was virtually no way for homeopaths to spread the good word about such practices as hydrotherapy, botanical herbal treatments, or the benefits of massage—especially in the face of impressive medical and chemical breakthroughs in allopathic medicine. Chemical and drug companies had—and continue to have—a major financial stake in the promotion of allopathic medications and treatments; as a result, natural remedies have been brushed aside in a storm of advertising and promotion on the part of those larger drug companies and the allopathic practitioners who have advocated them.

Even the earliest homeopaths recognized the importance of regulationg one's lifestyle as a highly important, controllable aspect of good health. Whether you are suffering from a medical condition or simply trying to improve the quality of your health, chances are you can feel better almost immediately by reducing your stress level. Learning to relax takes some time and effort, but the results of stress reduction benefit your cardiovascular system and your general sense of wellness. While most people need to work hard to accomplish goals at work, learning to take personal time to unwind and reflect should also be a priority. One method of learning to relax is biofeedback, which has proven helpful to patients with headaches, sore muscles, asthma complications, and stress-related problems. Hypnosis can induce a deeper contact with one's emotional life, resulting in the exposure of buried fears and conflicts and relief from repressions buried deep within the psyche. Massage methods such as reflexology and Swedish massage work miracles for relaxing tight muscles and loosening stiff necks that have been caused by hunching over a keyboard or spending long hours behind a desk. You will read about these and many other relaxation techniques in the *Physicians' Guides to Healing*.

Once you have mastered the art of relaxation, you will find it easier to make some more positive lifestyle changes. For instance, there's no time like the present if you've been intending to quit smoking or get in shape. Take a long walk. Make time to play outdoors with your children. Choose fresh fruit for dessert instead of pie. Use the stairs instead of the elevator. Wake up a few minutes early each morning to do some simple stretching. Physical activity will do a world of good and will make it much easier to change other bad habits into good ones. The small decisions you are faced with every day can turn into a set of healthy choices. Some alternative practitioners advocate hypnosis to correct behavioral difficulties such as smoking, overeating, and insomnia. Living an active, happy lifestyle free of harmful habits is one of the integral components of good health and a sense of overall vigor and vitality.

Besides lifestyle, one major element of health maintenance centers on diet and nutrition: a great deal of metabolic balance and general health depends on what foods we choose to put into our bodies. Nutrition was an inexact science until quite recently in this century. Nobody, including physicians and researchers, knew for certain what our bodies needed to subsist and flourish. The discovery of the existence of vitamins in the late nineteenth century prompted the theory that our bodies need three main types of nutrients to survive: food that builds and repairs tissue, food that can be burned for energy (calories), and food that regulates essential bodily functions.

For obvious reasons, both allopathic and alternative practitioners stress the importance of good diet. Feeding our bodies the wrong foods can promote cardiovascular disease, digestive stress, and general malaise. The government has developed a set of guidelines for proper nourishment and categorized them according to four major food groups: meat, vegetables, fruit, and dairy. Until the 1980s, a "balanced diet" consisted of equal amounts of each of these food groups, with an almost equal emphasis on meats and dairy products. While traditional medicine was inadvertently preaching this high-cholesterol, high-fat diet to the American public, holistic practitioners were advocating and enjoying the well-kept secret of vegetarianism and macrobiotics. To holistics, a balanced diet is one in which vegetables and grains prevail.

Nowadays the government guidelines for nutritional health have shifted away from the "four food group" grid in favor of a "food pyramid" in which the largest proportion of daily sustenance should be eaten from the grains category. The second largest category is fruits and vegetables. Then, smaller amounts of meat and poultry should be consumed, with the smallest daily servings in dairy and fats, oils, and sweets. There are more vegetarians—people who eat no red meat—and vegans—vegetarians who eat no animal products whatsoever, including eggs, cheese, and seafood—now than ever before; many people have discovered the benefits of eating low-fat and high-energy foods such as pasta, whole grains, and green leafy vegetables.

Another popular alternative approach to healing is chiropractic care, which is concerned with the relationship of the spinal column and the musculoskeletal structures of the body to the nervous system. The word "chiropractic" was derived from the Greek terms *cheir* (hand) and *praktikos* (practical). The main goal of chiropractic care is to help the body do its job. By correcting vertebral alignment, chiropractors minimize or eliminate interference to the normal flow of nerve energy throughout the body. This allows the body to repair its own systems and maintain good health without the use of drugs, surgery, or otherwise invasive medical procedures.

Chiropractic was conceived in an office building in Davenport, Iowa, in 1895. Its founder, Daniel David Palmer, noticed a bump on the spinal column of a janitor who, seventeen years earlier, had become suddenly and completely deaf when he had bent under a stairwell to reach for some cleaning supplies and had heard a prominent "snap." That noise was the last thing the man had heard for almost two decades. That is, until Daniel David Palmer pressed carefully on the janitor's spinal bump and immediately restored normal hearing to the deaf man. With one firm jolt, chiropractic treatment had been born.

Chiropractic health care is now performed by licensed practitioners in all fifty states. Common conditions treated by chiropractic include headaches, neck pain, bronchial asthma, stress, nervous disorders, gastrointestinal disorders, respiratory conditions, strains, arthritis, and migraine headaches. A chiropractic adjustment is a rapid, precise force (referred to as dynamic thrust) to a specific point on the vertebra. When applied properly, it removes nerve interference and induces the body to respond with an appropriate healing reaction. A chiropractic manipulation is a nonspecific procedure that resets bones, increases range of movement, and realigns joint structure. Some chiropractors also offer such services as acupressure, nutrition counseling, herbal care and homeopathic treatments.

Members of the health care community have come to recognize that there is a place for alternative approaches such as chiropractic care, the alteration of nutritional choices, and reevaluation of lifestyles in our health-conscious society. Such alternative treatments as relaxation therapy, biofeedback, massage, nutritional and vitamin supplements, low-stress lifestyles, and hydrotherapy are now being prescribed by allopathic practitioners not only as preventive strategies, but as treatments for health disorders and conditions that already exist. For the active, overworked people of the 1990s, the wealth of new options available to patients and practitioners—thanks to the wider acceptance of homeopathy—have been embraced as welcome additions to the old, traditional set of choices. Consult your volumes in the *Physicians' Guides to Healing* series for a comprehensive introduction to the world of complementary medicine and for reliable, accurate answers to all your health-related questions.

## THE PHYSICIANS' GUIDES TO HEALING

While homeopathy has been dismissed as "fringe" in the past and traditional medicine has prevailed, the past two decades have witnessed a movement back toward more natural and less invasive medical procedures. The benefits of both types of medicine are invaluable to complementary medical practitioners who treat patients with every disorder—from strokes and hypertension to hernias and ulcers; from hemorrhoids and rheumatoid arthritis to sprained joints; from urinary tract infections to menopausal discomfort, myocardial infarction, and seasonal hay fever. Who decides if you should use traditional treatments or alternative therapies? Is it necessary to choose between the two contrasting approaches, or can you safely combine them? How do you let your physician know your preferences? Is it possible for you to work as a team with your physician to determine how your symptoms should be treated, how your pain should be managed, and how long-term health may be maintained? The answers to all these questions, and many more, are readily available in each volume of the *Physicians' Guides to Healing* series.

# CHAPTER 1

---

# Introduction to Joint Disorders

There are more than one hundred joints in the human skeleton, which work together with the bones and muscles to provide a framework that supports the body and allows for flexible movement. From the earliest reach by an inquisitive toddler to the million-dollar moves of an NBA star, it is the joints that are relied upon for walking, running and lifting as well as activities such as talking, writing and chewing.

A disorder of the joints can be painful and sudden, as in a dislocated shoulder. Or it can be gradual and nearly painless, as are many forms of arthritis that can exist without any recognizable symptoms and be completely unknown to a patient until discovered on an X ray.

In the course of a lifetime, it is nearly impossible to avoid some occurrence of a joint disorder. With participation in competitive and recreational sports by people of all ages becoming more popular than ever, the likelihood of a strained, sprained, or dislocated joint is greater than ever before. More and more people are living longer and longer, and already it has been estimated that at least 80 percent of the population over the age of sixty-five already has arthritis to some degree.

In this volume of the *Physicians' Guides to Healing* series, the focus is on the most common maladies and problems that are likely to affect the body's joints. Although disorders of the joints are virtually never of a life-threatening nature, nagging pain and a high degree of discomfort are quite often present, so both traditional and natural techniques for lessening or eliminating pain have warranted an important place in each chapter. Additionally, ways of actually preventing or lessening the chances of contracting certain joint disorders are described.

The principle of integrating traditional and natural approaches to health care is particularly appropriate in dealing with problems of the joints. Many joint disorders have intense and acute stages of often very painful symptoms. For example, in the case of a chronic joint disorder such a rheumatoid arthritis, combining a traditional procedure that is designed to reduce the extent of damage with a natural therapy that will lessen the painful symptoms can make for an effective treatment plan.

Throughout this volume, the symptoms and causes of various joint disorders will be described, along with recommended choices of treatment, both traditional and alternative, as well as methods of prevention.

In chapter 2, the confusing and complicated disorder of temporomandibular joint disorder, known as TMD, is explored. Although many medical experts disagree as to whether TMD is more of a muscle-and-ligament problem than an affliction of the joints, there is no doubt as to the painful symptoms of this ailment, which affect the jaw joint, nearby muscles and sometimes the entire facial area.

The reduction of TMD pain is the most urgent aspect of this disorder, and many traditional and alternative methods are described. Just as important for TMD sufferers, however, is learning how to stop it from occurring, and a number of preventive techniques are explored.

Chapter 3 focuses on osteoarthritis, the most common of the one hundred varieties of arthritis, which afflicts more than sixteen million people in the U.S. Since osteoarthritis develops over a period of years, with the symptoms usually not recognized until after sufferers have reached the age of fifty, it's considered an "old age" disease. Given the fact that virtually everyone over the age of sixty-five can expect to have some degree of osteoarthritis, it makes good sense for everyone to learn about this disease.

There are some special challenges that are related to osteoarthritis, including the typically recurrent outbreaks of symptoms that alternate with periods of remission. There has also been a proliferation of unscrupulous and deceptive sales pitches for an astonishing variety of unproved and even dangerous so-called remedies. At the same time, numerous alternative treatments for osteoarthritis have been shown to be effective and many of them are described in the chapter.

Rheumatoid arthritis, the most common form of inflammatory arthritis, is examined in chapter 4. Unlike osteoarthritis, rheumatoid arthritis afflicts people long before age fifty, usually beginning between the ages of twenty and forty-five. Another way in which rheumatoid arthritis differs from osteoarthritis is that it is systemic, causing symptoms in other organs in the body.

Like osteoarthritis, rheumatoid arthritis alternates periods of remission with periods of flare-up. There is no cure as yet for rheumatoid arthritis, so keeping joint damage to a minimum and managing the painful symptoms over many years present formidable challenges. Some of the most effective anti-inflammatory drugs have severe and even alarming side effects, so that being able to find natural, alternative treatments for pain relief is a important concern.

Since finding the treatment regimens that are most effective and most comfortable is an individual decision, numerous therapeutic approaches, both traditional and alternative, for managing rheumatoid arthritis are detailed in this chapter.

In chapter 5, the mystifying and disconcerting ailment called Lyme disease is spotlighted. Public awareness of this infectious disease, which is caused by the bite of a tiny tick, has increased dramatically following several years of vigorous public education by the Center for Disease Control.

Yet the complex nature of Lyme disease, with more than forty separate recognizable symptoms, a number of stages that can last for many years, and the possibility of this condition being mistaken for any one of nearly two hundred other ailments, results in many cases not being diagnosed promptly.

In this chapter, you'll learn about the advances in testing procedures, treatment options, locales where infectious ticks are likely to be found, and techniques for preventing Lyme disease.

Chapter 6 details the painful condition of bursitis, which can occur in the shoulder, hip, elbow, wrist, heels, knees, and even the base of the big toe. Bursitis is usually the result of repetitive movements, especially in an awkward position or following a prolonged, excessive pressure. After several days of rather intense pain, followed by ten days of continued healing, the condition subsides.

Although not a serious condition, bursitis can result in permanent impairment if not treated properly. Careful adherence to treatment guidelines is important, and the appropriate procedures are described in this chapter.

Gout, the legendary disease of the rich and the royal, is the subject of chapter 7. More than one million people in the U.S. suffer from this condition, with at least 90 percent of those being men over forty, who are usually overweight and often have a family history of the disease.

There are three major concerns about gout, which constitute the main focus of the chapter: having the condition positively confirmed; arriving at effective treatment of the pain and inflammation; and finding a strategy for minimizing the possibility of future attacks.

Sprains and dislocations, covered in chapter 8, are traumatic injuries to the joints that can range in severity from very mild to very serious. It's important to learn how to evaluate the seriousness of an injury as well as to know the basic emergency and first-aid procedures that should be followed. Along with such information, the chapter also includes a variety of traditional and alternative techniques for the long-term healing and rehabilitation of sprains and dislocations.

In chapter 9, the chronic stiff-back condition that is known as inflammatory back pain, or ankylosing spondylitis, is described. This disease involves a form of inflammatory arthritis that affects joints of the spine and the sacroiliac joints. As the inflammation subsides, bone grows out from both sides of the joint, eventually surrounding the joint completely, thereby causing it to stiffen.

Symptoms of inflammatory back pain usually begin in early adulthood or adolescence and are often ignored because of widespread back pain that is caused by growing pains or during physical activities. Information in the chapter includes both traditional and alternative ways to relieve the symptoms and restore spinal mobility, as well as ways to pursue a normal occupational and social life.

Bunions are the topic of chapter 10, where the causes and recommended cures are outlined. Resulting from the excessive pronation of an improper walking pattern, bunions are more likely to occur in women than in men.

Having a genetic tendency for foot problems and wearing ill-fitting footwear contribute to the escalation of a bunion into a chronic deformity. Ways of rethinking the selection and sizing of footwear are stressed in the chapter, which also suggests methods for minimizing pain and reducing inflammation.

Chapter 11 offers a look at the problems of repetitive motion injury, specifically that of carpal tunnel syndrome. Hands and wrists are the most common areas in which symptoms of carpal tunnel syndrome are experienced, although the condition can affect the entire upper extremity, including not only the hand, wrist, and forearm, but also the upper arm, upper back, neck and shoulder.

Ways of treating carpal tunnel syndrome and regaining previous mobility are the main focus of this chapter, along with ideas for preventing its appearance or reappearance.

Throughout this guide, the sheer number and variety of traditional and alternative therapeutic options that are described for treating conditions of the joints offer a great deal of choice in therapies. A common thread in many of these treatments is the basic orientation to a healthy lifestyle, especially in an ongoing emphasis on proper nutrition and exercise.

In becoming more involved and ultimately responsible for the treatment plan of a disorder, a patient must be willing to invest time and effort in studying the details of the condition, learning about the treatments that are available, and evaluating the options.

# CHAPTER 2

_____

# Temporomandibular Joint Disorder

"Lips together, teeth apart" is a familiar treatment mantra for millions of Americans who suffer from temporomandibular joint syndrome. The affected joint is located where the sides of the lower jaw are attached to the skull, although the name is used to describe a group of painful ailments that affect the jaw joint, muscles and the entire facial area.

Although an estimated one in three persons suffers from some degree of temporomandibular joint disorder, called TMD (formerly known as TMJ), the syndrome is controversial, confusing, and complicated. TMD is the object of controversy because some medical professionals argue that it should be classified as a muscle-and-ligament problem while others believe that it is correctly categorized as an affliction of the bone and cartilage. The disorder is confusing because no one is really certain about what actually causes it. Stress, misaligned teeth, whiplash, growth problems, arthritis, clenching and grinding of the teeth, and a blow to the jaw are all possibilities. Complicating matters even more is that the various painful symptoms associated with TMD take many forms, going well beyond the jaw region.

The most common symptom of TMD is the pain or swelling in the jaw or at the temporomandibular joints, where both sides of the lower jaw are attached to the skull. Other symptoms include clicking, popping, or scraping noises when opening or closing the jaw; difficulty in opening and closing the jaw; the temporary locking of the jaw into place; a tenderness of the muscles used for chewing; unexplained muscle aches in the neck, shoulders or upper back; persistent migrainelike headaches; pain behind the eyes; earaches; stiff neck; stuffiness in the nasal passages; pain in the back teeth; facial pain. Even sinuslike problems, diminished hearing, and ringing in the ears are considered symptoms of TMD.

There are different degrees in the level of pain that is encountered with TMD. More than half of the people with symptoms do not find them severe enough to seek treatment. For others, however, the pain is constant and excruciating. Many people who do seek medical treatment are experiencing severe headaches or finding that it is too painful even to open their mouth or brush their teeth.

In some instances, the problem can be felt in the actual temporomandibular joint while in others, the pain is in the muscles of the jaw. The temporomandibular joint itself can be located by putting your finger in front of your ear, then opening and closing the mouth. The movable part that you feel is called a condyle, the round-tipped end of the lower jawbone. When the mouth is closed, the condyle normally rests in the temporomandibular joint. A cushion of cartilage allows the condyle to move inside the joint like a ball bearing.

When the pain is not emanating from the joint, it's likely coming from one of the muscles that is responsible for opening and closing the mouth. To get an idea of how long and powerful the muscle is, place your fingers on the temple muscles right behind your eyes and then bite down tightly. You will be able to feel the tightening of the temple muscle, which covers most of each side of the head.

The prolonged grinding of teeth or clenching of the jaw is considered by specialists to be a primary cause of TMD. As a result, over a period of time the muscles that control the temporomandibular joints develop nodules that act as trigger points and produce the symptoms of TMD when they are aggravated. For many people, this grinding or clenching is a conscious way of dealing with many levels of stress in their lives. For others, the grinding occurs at night and they are not aware of it.

In addition to grinding and clenching, other damaging habits are believed to cause or contribute to TMD. Some of these habits include prolonged and intense biting down on a pencil or pipe; chewing on hard candies or ice; nail biting; biting on cheeks or the tongue. Even poor posture, such as sitting for long hours at a desk with the jaw jutting out, can be a contributing cause. Obviously, the end result of any of these habits will be dependent on the intensity and duration of the activity.

Also considered to be a major cause of TMD is a malocclusion of the jaw, the result of teeth not fitting together properly. This can be either a case of poor alignment when the mouth is closed or a side-to-side movement of the bottom jaw. After a time, the muscles in the jaw work to compensate for this improper biting relationship, causing pain and the other symptoms of TMD. There are many people, however, who can go through life with a malocclusion of the jaw and never have any symptoms of TMD or even be aware that their teeth aren't aligned properly.

In addition to existing structural conditions, there are unforeseen situations that can cause malocclusion problems, including a missing tooth that causes shifting of other teeth; a new filling that alters the way in which the previous components functioned; and an addition of bridgework to the mouth.

TMD can also be the result of a trauma such as a punch in the jaw or whiplash. In some rare cases, TMD occurs as the result of arthritis.

If you experience persistent headaches, neck and back pain, or stuffiness or swelling of your sinus area that doesn't respond to sinus treatments, you might be affected with TMD. A preliminary test that you can do yourself is to feel your temples and then clench your jaw. The muscle will tense up under your fingers at the temples. Keeping your fingers there, relax the jaw and press down on those muscles. If you feel severe pain and tenderness, TMD may be the cause. Another self-test is to put the tips of your little fingers into your ears, pressing them forward toward the front of the ears while opening and closing your mouth. If you can feel the head of your jawbone pushing against your fingers, you might have TMD.

The next step would be to visit your dentist, and possibly a doctor as well, for a confirmation of the diagnosis. Although such tests as X rays, computed tomography (CT) scans, or magnetic resonance imaging (MRI) can be performed, people with TMD often will not show abnormalities. So you must rely mostly on a diagnosis that is based on a description of your symptoms and a physical examination.

That's why it is important to consult with a specialist who is knowledgeable about TMD.

## Traditional Treatments

*Mouth guard*   Using a removable plastic or rubber mold known as a mouth guard, which is horseshoe-shaped and designed to separate the surfaces of the teeth, can prevent the clenching of the jaw or the grinding together of the teeth. This appliance is meant to be worn at night, and is especially useful for those patients for whom tooth grinding does not occur during the day and who are not aware of their teeth grinding at night. Studies have shown that mouth guards eliminate 70 to 80 percent of the symptoms of clenching and grinding.

*Bite plate*   Similar to a mouth guard, a bite plate is a removable appliance that is designed to prevent clenching and grinding by separating the biting surfaces of the teeth. It is worn during the day and taken out for meals.

*Surgical repair*   The surgical repair of damaged joint tissues and bone defects is a procedure for TMD patients that is rarely recommended nowadays and which should only be undertaken as a last resort because there is a serious risk of severe complications, including facial paralysis. Such surgery should be considered only after it has been determined that it is absolutely necessary and there are no alternatives. Even then, a number of expert opinions should be solicited. Such a procedure may involve a recontouring of the articular bone or a repair of displaced disks.

*Nonprescriptive pain relievers*   Aspirin or acetaminophen are nonprescriptive pain relievers that can offer temporary relief from discomfort, reduce inflammation, and allow the patient to relax and untense the jaw muscles.

*Tranquilizers*  Sometimes tranquilizers are prescribed to relax the jaw muscles.

*Corticosteroids*  Injections of corticosteroids into the temporomandibular joints can reduce severe inflammation.

## Alternative Treatments

*Acupressure*  An effective technique to combat the pain of TMD is acupressure, pressing both the points near the jaw area, called the St 6 points using the middle finger. Press these points for about one minute, two or three times a day. You can locate the points by clenching your back teeth and feeling for the muscles that bulge between the upper and lower jaw, near the jaw area.

*Acupuncture*  An acupuncturist will recommend techniques not only for the specific relief from the pain symptoms of TMD but also as a way of redirecting the energy flow that may be contributing to the underlying problem.

*The Alexander Technique*  Useful in the treatment of TMD is the Alexander Technique because it stresses proper alignment of the neck and back. Since the muscles of the neck control the muscles in the jaw, misuse of the neck muscles can affect the jaw and aggravate any existing condition. Realignment and proper, natural posture through training in the Alexander Technique has been shown to be very beneficial for that reason.

*Biofeedback*  Through the use of biofeedback training, a patient may be able to gain voluntary control over certain of the body's reactions to stress. In the case of TMD, the emphasis is on trying to lessen contractions in the muscles of the jaw, neck and shoulder in reaction to stress and anxiety. Some studies have shown that nearly 70 percent of those who undergo biofeedback training eliminate their clenching and grinding habits.

*Improved habits*    It has been shown in many cases to be remarkably effective when bad habits that cause or acerbate TMD are eliminated, especially among patients who exercise the commitment and discipline required. For example, people who previously experienced frequent periods of prolonged yawning have been able to stifle the yawns by placing a fist under the chin. Those people who have the habit of clenching their teeth in moments of stress or emotion have learned to eliminate that habit by using the "lips together, teeth apart" method. This consists of placing the tongue behind the top front teeth, so that it rests against the roof of the mouth. This position not only separates the top and bottom teeth, it also relaxes the jaw.

Cradling the phone between the shoulder and the chin is also a habit that encourages TMD, and it should be consciously eliminated. For heavy phone users who need to keep their hands free, a headset should be substituted for a receiver.

Another bad habit that promotes TMD is to lie flat on one's back with the head propped up at a sharp angle with a pillow or cushion, which many people do when watching television or reading. Also, a person who spends long periods of time with the chin cupped in hands is promoting or aggravating TMD and needs to eliminate that posture.

*Chiropractic*    Adjustment of the vertebrae through chiropractic can be useful in treating TMD because the temporomandibular joint is structurally involved in the cervical spine. When the base cause of TMD is associated with spinal alignment, chiropractic treatment can have lasting effects. If TMD is linked to a dental cause, chiropractic treatment can at least be helpful in alleviating the symptoms of the ailment.

*Cognitive therapy*    The technique of cognitive therapy focuses on how to look differently at a situation, with the goal of having more positive perceptions that will produce more positive emotional responses. For example, in dealing with the painful symptoms of TMD, one could react with great despair, immediately thinking how awful and uncomfortable and possibly unbearable it would be. Or, using skills of cognitive therapy, at the first sign of pain, one can begin to think immediately of trying out one of the methods of pain reduction, looking forward to mastering the problem and being in command. Additionally, cognitive therapy can be applied to the bigger picture, where the kinds of problems that create stress and, in turn, symptoms of TMD, instead become challenges to be handled with relish.

*Food therapy*    Some researchers believe that food has a relevance to TMD problems. If a person has a history of food allergies, any foods that might be considered to have the possibility of causing a reaction should be eliminated from the diet. Additionally, when the jaw is tender or aches, a soft diet is preferable. Avoid raw vegetables and chewy foods like bagels. Some specialists in treating TMD believe that after a flare-up in the jaw muscles, a diet of soft foods should be pursued for twelve weeks, eliminating everything that is chewy, crunchy or hard, even if some relief is felt after only a few days because not only the obvious symptoms but the entire condition is likely to be improved.

It is thought that people who consume a great deal of caffeine are likely to clench their jaws far more frequently than people who do not have caffeine in their diets. Also, low blood sugar is suspected of contributing to more frequent teeth clenching, so it's important for people who have hypoglycemia to maintain their diets and be vigilant about avoiding the consumption of sugar.

*Herbal treatment*   Herbs can be used to reduce the pain and discomfort of TMD. Commonly used are white willow bark, passion flower, hops and valerian. There are various formulations of these herbs that are recommended for treatment, with a variety of different recipes prescribed by herbalists.

*Hydrotherapy*   One way to relieve the pain of TMD is through hydrotherapy, using either heat or cold, depending on the type of pain that is involved. A moist heat pad, applied for fifteen minutes three or four times a day, increases the blood flow and loosens tense muscles when the pain is achy. A cloth wrung out in very warm water or a moist heat pack wrapped in a towel can be used.

When the TMD pain is experienced in hard spasms or is the result of a forceful blow to the jaw, cold therapy is prescribed instead of heat. Put an ice bag against the area for ten minutes, then remove it for ten minutes; repeat the process for an hour. Be sure the bag is wrapped in a towel to protect the skin from frostbite or burn.

*Hypnosis*   There are two ways in which hypnosis can be beneficial in the treatment of TMD. First, hypnosis can be administered to a patient or self-applied as a way to combat the painful symptoms. A trance is utilized to instruct the patient to not feel any pain. When successful, the relief from pain will last for some time after the session. A second way to use hypnosis is as a method to eliminate the habits that can cause or aggravate the condition. Through hypnotic techniques, a patient can be programmed to stop teeth grinding or clenching.

**Guided imagery**   Techniques that utilize the power of the mind to produce a positive response in the body can be a force to counteract tense muscles. As soon as muscles in the jaw, neck or shoulder begin to tense, guided imagery can be used to visualize a tranquil, floating state of pure relaxation that should reverse the beginning of tenseness.

**Massage**   The use of massage techniques on the jaw muscles helps to lessen the pain of muscle tension that accompanies TMD. One set of muscles to focus on is situated at the back of the jaw, away from the chin. These muscles can be located by clenching the teeth and feeling for the muscles with the fingers: left fingers on the left side of the jaw, right fingers on the right side. Once the muscles are located, unclench the teeth and rub the muscles with small, firm circular strokes until the tensions release. It's also helpful to press into the muscles with the fingertips and hold for ten to fifteen seconds.

There's a second set of jaw muscles, which can be located by clenching the teeth and touching the scalp in front of the tops of the ears. After unclenching the teeth, use the same techniques as before to rub and press these muscles. This kind of massage should be done for about ten minutes once a day or in the case of acute pain, two or three times a day.

**Nutritional supplements**   Considered helpful in fighting TMD are the nutritional supplements of calcium and pantothenic acid. Nutrition specialists recommend 1,200 mg of calcium daily, taken at bedtime, and 200 mg of pantothenic acid daily, in addition to any regular vitamin supplements. Also recommended is 100 mg of vitamin B complex, three times daily; 60 mg of coenzyme Q daily; 500 mg of L-Tyrosine daily; 50 mg of vitamin $B_6$ and vitamin C daily; a multivitamin daily.

***Relaxation techniques*** One method recommended for relieving TMD pain is called stretched-based relaxation. With this method, you push up the eyebrows with your index fingers and push down on your cheeks with your thumbs and hold the position for about ten seconds. Then release and let the muscles around the eyes relax. After a minute of relaxing, let the head slowly drop toward the right shoulder for about ten seconds. Then slowly drop the head toward the left should for another ten seconds. Be sure not to raise the chin, to prevent overextension of the head-and-neck muscles.

***Sleep position*** Sleeping on the side or stomach puts pressure on one side of the jaw, which causes TMD pain. Instead, it's important to sleep on one's back. This isn't natural or easy for many people, but there are some aids that can be of assistance. One approach is to place under the neck a thin towel, rolled up, rather than a pillow. Have another towel placed under the back and a pillow under the knees.

## Combined Treatments

In recent years, both the medical and dental communities have expressed a preference for conservative, noninvasive treatments for TMD. The risk of severe complications, especially from infections, has been a major factor in their stance. Also, many of the factors that trigger TMD are related to habits of the patient that can be self-corrected, and the natural and alternative techniques that emphasize the relationship between mind and healing can play an important and beneficial role.

Even when a traditional method such as a mouth guard is being used for treating TMD, a patient ought to be combining techniques with it such as the elimination of clenching and grinding, which is a major factor aggravating the condition.

There are a great number of methods for reducing stress and gaining a relaxed state. It's a good idea for a person to experiment and try many of them until the most effective, most enjoyable approach is found.

Table 1

# TREATMENTS FOR TEMPOROMANDIBULAR JOINT DISORDER

| Traditional | Alternative |
|---|---|
| *Tooth reshaping* | *Acupressure* <br> St 6 points |
| *Mouth guard* <br> worn at night | *Acupuncture* |
| *Bite plate* <br> worn in daytime | *Alexander Technique* |
| | *Biofeedback training* |
| *Surgical repair* <br> recontouring of articular bone; repair of disks, joint tissues | *Improved habits* |
| | *Chiropractic medicine* |
| | *Cognitive therapy* |
| | *Food therapy* |
| *Nonprescriptive pain relievers* <br> aspirin; acetaminophen | *Herbal treatment* <br> white willow bark; passion flower; hops; valerian |
| *Tranquilizers* <br> ask physician | *Hydrotherapy* <br> heat; cold |
| *Corticosteroids* <br> ask physician | *Hypnosis* |
| | *Guided imagery* |
| | *Massage* |
| | *Nutritional supplements* <br> calcium; pantothenic acid; vitamin supplements |
| | *Relaxation techniques* |
| | *Sleep position* |

# CHAPTER 3

---

# Osteoarthritis

**B**y the age of sixty-five, virtually everyone can expect to have some degree of osteoarthritis, the form of arthritis that slowly wears away the cartilage covering the ends of the joints and results in a deterioration of the cushioning between bones. Damage is gradual, developing over a period of years, which is one reason why the disease is often called a degenerative joint disease or the "wear and tear" arthritis. As the bones rub against each other, uneven outgrowths called osteophytes or spurs begin to form that may, in turn, grind against each other. This process causes various degrees of pain and loss of mobility.

More than sixteen million people in the U.S. have osteoarthritis, the most common of the one hundred varieties of arthritis. Many people are not even aware that the disease is present because they do not experience pain or other symptoms. In fact, while most people over sixty will show signs of osteoarthritis on an X ray, only about a third of them have experienced any symptoms. For others, however, there can be severe pain and the loss of function.

Typical symptoms of osteoarthritis are episodes of pain and stiffness, which occur at intervals of months or sometimes years. Inflammation can also be present, although redness and warmth are not commonly seen with osteoarthritis. When they are, it's the result of cartilage fragments that infiltrate the joint. Unlike rheumatoid arthritis, which is an inflammatory disease that invades other parts of the body, osteoarthritis is not systemic. Therefore, symptoms like malaise, fever and fatigue generally do not occur.

Since the first symptoms of osteoarthritis usually begin to appear during the same time that signs of aging are also starting to occur, the signs often are not recognized as being associated with the early stages of osteoarthritis.

Medical experts long believed that osteoarthritis was simply and entirely an inevitable result of the aging process. It is certainly true that the disease is seen most often in middle-aged and older people, rarely appearing before the age of forty. However, a few years ago scientific evidence was established that there is a genetic defect that contributes to the occurrence of osteoarthritis in the hands. The presence of the gene results in a weakening of the protein whose job it is to strengthen the cartilage that cushions the joints. Also, trauma from an injury, such as a blow to a joint that occurs during an athletic injury, can result in the formation of osteoarthritis in that joint many years later. There is also evidence that years of a repeated motion, such as sewing or weaving, can result in osteoarthritis in the fingers.

Some researchers believe that various chemical reactions of the body that control the metabolism of cartilage in the joint can operate improperly and harm the cartilage, which could result eventually in osteoarthritis. Some day, it may be possible for persons from families with osteoarthritis to be tested for the defective gene. They might be able to delay or even prevent the onset of osteoarthritis by avoiding activities that irritate joints.

Typically, osteoarthritis occurs in only three locations: the fingers, the spine and the weight-bearing joints, namely the hips, knees or feet. Unlike rheumatoid arthritis, which frequently attacks many joints, most people will have the symptoms of osteoarthritis in just one place. However, it is possible for osteoarthritis to attack two or even all three locations, at the same time or at different times.

Even when osteoarthritis is limited to a single location, the affected joint can cause serious disruption to the smooth workings of the entire body. Muscles that are located away from the joint may begin to tighten in order to avoid pain or to protect the afflicted joint, while unaffected joints may begin working overtime to make up for any deficiencies. When knee cartilage has been seriously depleted, the entire lower leg may eventually be deformed.

Among all arthritis patients, about 25 percent have serious arthritic problems with their hands and wrists. Osteoarthritis of the hand increases with age, so that by age seventy-five, fully 85 percent of the population have some evidence of the condition. The gnarled appearance of arthritic fingers is caused by the bony knobs that enlarge the finger joints. These knobs, called nodes or nodules, usually appear spontaneously but can be caused by injury.

Nearly 90 percent of cases of nodal osteoarthritis, as it is often called, afflict women over the age of forty-five. It is believed to be a hereditary condition. Nodes most often begin prominently in just one finger but can involve all of the finger to some degree. While there can be tenderness, stiffness and pain with nodes, there is little chance of any real disability. There are certain activities, such as turning handles or opening jars, that may become clumsy or slightly painful, however.

Spinal osteoarthritis, especially when it affects the neck and lumbar spine, is fairly common, although not always to the extent of causing any clinical symptoms. Osteoarthritis can develop in the joints that connect the upper part of the spine as well as in the joints of the spine itself. The bony outgrowths, or osteophytes, can be detected by X ray but usually don't change a person's appearance. Many researchers believe that lifestyle habits, including prolonged sitting, cigarette smoking, consumption of alcohol, and weight gain, contribute to the onset of spinal osteoarthritis. However, for the most part the primary cause is not known.

The knees, hips and feet are where osteoarthritis strikes with the most damaging results because they support the weight of the entire body. These weight-bearing joints are most susceptible to osteoarthritis after either long-term exposure to heavy-lifting occupations, such as mining, or the aggravation of an injury in a contact sport like football. Not surprisingly, then, osteoarthritis in the knees, hips, and feet occurs more frequently in men than in women.

Although the hip joint cannot be readily felt, being located about four inches within the groin, advanced osteoarthritis of the hip can be a severely disabling condition. In fact, before the development of joint replacement surgery, a diseased hip meant life in a wheelchair or on crutches. Today, more than one hundred fifteen thousand hips are replaced in the U.S. every year, with nearly 95 percent of these patients experiencing good to excellent results.

Fortunately, while the hip joints of virtually all older persons show signs of wear, the majority do not develop serious osteoarthritis. The initial pain of very mild osteoarthritis can be significant, however, leading patients to incorrectly suspect a far worse condition. When there is advanced osteoarthritis of the hip, developing over many years, a patient is usually dealing with constant pain, a decrease in function, and often an intolerance for anti-inflammatory drugs. This is the point at which surgical replacement of the joint becomes a serious consideration.

The knee is undoubtedly the most complicated joint in the body, both in its design and function. It can fold upon itself, rotate, and lock into place. Despite its flexibility, however, the knee is a vulnerable area because it has little inherent stability and must rely on the ligaments and muscles that surround it. So, whenever those ligaments or muscles are injured, the knee becomes even more unstable and vulnerable.

As in other joints, it is not known just what triggers osteoarthritis of the knee. Factors that are considered most likely include poor alignment, such as being bowlegged or knock-kneed, damaged ligaments or traumatic injuries that took place many years before. A knee injury that is not correctly treated at the time the joint was injured becomes a nagging condition that, in time, eventually becomes a serious case of osteoarthritis.

In the past twenty years, there has been considerable advancement in surgical procedures that can alleviate afflicted knees. For example, the use of a surgical instrument, the arthroscope, enables surgeons to more readily examine the interior of the knee and make small repairs. Also important is the development of techniques for the partial and total replacement of the knee surfaces for severely damaged knee joints.

## Traditional Treatments

Although there is no cure yet for osteoarthritis, much progress has been made in its treatment, with a variety of effective methods that are widely used to reduce pain and to limit the disabling effects of the disease. Indeed, since there is such a large segment of the population that is coping with osteoarthritis and because there is a strong desire among all patients to find relief from its painful symptoms, the variety of available options is enormous, contributing to a great deal of confusion among osteoarthritis patients, who are liable to try almost any remedy in the hope of finding an effective solution. Many of these treatments are harmless at best while others that might be the most appropriate are not widely known.

Official recommendations for the treatment of osteoarthritis had never been issued until 1995, when the American College of Rheumatology released the first-ever guidelines for the medical management of two forms of osteoarthritis; those affecting the knee and the hip. The suggestions include the use of simple analgesics for relief of pain; regular exercise programs; weight reduction if overweight and the use of assisting devices such as elastic shoe laces, levers to turn faucets, and extended shoe horns.

It is important to stay up-to-date about treatment with information from reputable sources such as the Arthritis Foundation and the American College of Rheumatology, along with the recommendations of your physician. Osteoarthritis is an individual and long-term challenge for each patient, and is best approached with a treatment plan that is individual in its design, reflecting the needs and concerns of the individual. Since you will need to follow a treatment plan for the rest of your life, you must be comfortable with it and be ready to make adjustments to keep it fresh and effective.

*Acetaminophens*  Over-the-counter analgesics that are called acetaminophens, such as Tylenol, act like aspirin in decreasing pain and lowering fever. However, an important advantage of an acetaminophen is that it does not irritate the stomach. The American College of Rheumatology considers acetaminophens to be the first choice for pain relief, far more desirable for treating the pain associated with osteoarthritis than nonsteroidal anti-inflammatory drugs (NSAIDs), which for many years have been a popular choice (see below). Since the pain from osteoarthritis, unlike rheumatoid arthritis, has very little to do with inflammation, NSAIDs are not really appropriate, especially since there are side effects associated with its continued use. The recommended dosage of acetaminophen is 4,000 mg daily. It is possible for some side effects to emerge after prolonged usage, however.

*Topical analgesics*    The use of topical analgesics such as methyl salicylate or capsaicin cream, applied directly to the affected joint, can be also be an effective way of relieving pain without the side effects of NSAIDs.

*Aspirin*    A widely used pain reliever for osteoarthritis is aspirin, probably because it is a proven remedy already familiar to most households. Caution is needed in using aspirin because excessive amounts can irritate the stomach and cause ringing in the ears, heartburn, nausea and even vomiting, diarrhea or gastrointestinal bleeding. The usual dosage is two tablets of 325 mg each, four times a day. There are many varieties of aspirin, including buffered, film-coated, enteric-coated and time-release, so you may want to try different versions to see if one offers a superior result.

*Nonsteroidal anti-inflammatory drugs (NSAIDs)*    Very popular in the treatment of arthritis are nonsteroidal anti-inflammatory drugs (NSAIDS), especially for rheumatoid arthritis, because NSAIDs not only relieve pain but also reduce inflammation. However, there are possible side effects, including upset stomach, heartburn, nausea, diarrhea, rash, weight gain, headache, drowsiness, dizziness, increased bleeding when cut, ear ringing, stomach ulcers, gastritis, bleeding ulcers, kidney problems and blood problems. There are over-the-counter NSAIDs known as ibuprofen, including Advil, Motrin and Nuprin, as well as more than a dozen types of NSAIDs that are available by prescription. An NSAID is not the most appropriate pain reliever for osteoarthritis since inflammation is a very limited element associated with the condition.

*Heat therapy*    An effective way of relieving the pain of osteoarthritis is through heat therapy, which relaxes the muscles around the affected joint, increases the blood flow and lessens the stiffness. Moist heat seems to work better than dry heat and can be gotten simply by taking a relaxing hot bath or, for a more localized treatment, applying a hot-water bottle. A whirlpool bath is both soothing and stimulating for many people. Also good for treating localized areas is a moist hot pack. One method of preparing a hot pack is to heat a wet towel in the microwave for two or three minutes at medium heat. At the drugstore there are also hot packs available that when activated will last for about one half hour. When using any hot compresses, be sure to protect your skin from burning by placing a cloth or towel over the area before applying the pack.

There are also special treatments in which different forms of energy are converted to deep, penetrating heat. Diathermy and ultrasound are commonly utilized methods of deep, penetrating heat. In diathermy treatments, short-wave radiation is transformed into deep heat. This method should not be used by patients who have metallic implants because the radiation tends to concentrate in metal. Before treatment, one must take care to remove all metallic jewelry and any clothing with metal fasteners. Ultrasound therapy utilizes high-energy sound waves, which convert to heat and can be delivered to the deeper joint areas. Along with improving joint movement, ultrasound treatment also warms injured tissue, relieves muscle tension and increases blood circulation.

*Cold treatments*  When there is intense pain, cold treatments are used to relieve inflamed joints. Since cold also acts as a local anesthetic, it can decrease muscle spasms and soothe muscle aches that come from holding muscles tightly to avoid pain. It is important that ice not be placed directly on the skin because that can cause frostbite or tissue damage. Wrapping ice cubes or even a bag of frozen vegetables in a towel are methods of creating simple ice packs. There are also instant, disposable cold packs that are chemically activated and last for about twenty minutes as well as reusable gel packs that are first frozen in the freezer before using. Don't apply cold packs for more than twenty minutes at a time because frostbite can occur after longer periods of time. It's all right for the area to become reddish and a little bit numb, but should it become white or blue, remove the cold pack immediately.

*Weight control*  An important aspect of an osteoarthritis treatment plan is weight control. The more excess weight that a person carries, the more stress and pressure are placed on the joint, which adds stress on the cartilage and increases pain and any swelling. Studies have shown that overweight persons with osteoarthritis may be able to reduce the level of painful symptoms by losing weight, while those without the disease are able to reduce the risk for developing it.

*Exercise*   An essential part of ongoing therapy for osteoarthritis is an exercise program, because inactivity can result in muscles becoming weaker and joints stiffening. Weak muscles are not able to support joints as well, while coordination and posture may also deteriorate. Not all exercise is appropriate for patients with osteoarthritis, however. Weight-bearing or high-impact activities such as running or basketball are likely to aggravate the condition. Ideal exercises include swimming, walking, stationary bicycling and cross-country skiing. Floor exercises are appropriate for arthritis in the back.

Quite possibly the single most pleasurable and beneficial activity for arthritis sufferers is exercise in a warm swimming pool. The buoyancy of the water reduces stress on the joints and makes exercise easier. Thanks to buoyancy, a person in a pool weighs only about 10 percent of normal "land" weight. Additionally, a warm swimming pool decreases pain and feels good. So-called aqua exercises will help to reduce pain and stiffness, increase muscle strength and improve flexibility and stamina. These aqua exercises consist of various waving, walking and bending motions performed in waist-high water, and they progress to patterns of aqua dance.

A special program of aquatic exercises is conducted by the Arthritis Foundation at various YMCAs and YWCAs throughout the United States. Any local chapter of the Arthritis Foundation can provide details about area programs. The foundation also sells a videotape that demonstrates a number of different pool exercises.

No matter what kind of exercise or activity you undertake, if you feel pain for two hours afterwards, you've done too much. It would then make sense to divide the activity into segments and reduce the intensity of the activity. The best time to exercise is when you feel the best—when the pain medication is most effective or after a hot bath. Always start slowly to avoid fatigue and muscle pain. After exercising vigorously, rest your joints until you feel completely recovered.

*Corticosteroids*   Prescription drugs called corticosteroids, which are modified forms of hormones made in the adrenal gland, are effective in reducing pain and inflammation. While steroids are not prescribed in oral form for osteoarthritis, they may occasionally be injected into an acutely inflamed weight-bearing joint such as the hip, knee or ankle. Most common among the twenty steroid drugs is prednisone. Since this drug actually may accelerate joint disease, a doctor will limit the number of injections to no more than two or three times a year, and usually only at times of extreme pain.

*Occupational therapy*   Techniques of occupational therapy can help to prevent loss of function and improve a person's ability to perform daily tasks when faced with limitations from osteoarthritis. Preserving energy and protecting joints are the key principles utilized to minimize fatigue, reduce stress on joints, reduce pain and increase performance. Patients are trained in alternate methods and the use of adaptive equipment for performing daily self-care and tasks at work, home and leisure.

A key premise in planning and managing activities is to alternate those that require substantial energy with those that are less strenuous. This technique will help to preserve energy and also to protect joints. Depending on the condition of a joint, a splint may be recommended to improve function, prevent contracture or shortening, provide stability and lessen pain.

It is a good idea to develop the habit of refraining from positions that promote misalignment or deformity of the joints. For example, when in the kitchen, stir with the thumb on top of the spoon as though holding an ice pick and make the circular motion with the shoulder instead of the hand. Refrain from leaning on your hands if you're standing against a railing. Try to avoid unnecessary wringing motions simply by letting washcloths dry or by using an electric rather than a handheld can opener. Always use the largest joint and strongest muscle available. Therefore, try to open doors with the power from the upper arm or even hip rather than from the fingers. When getting up from a sitting position, try to use the whole body to rise, avoiding pressure on the hip and knee joints. This involves sliding forward as far as possible, then leaning forward and swinging up, pushing off with forearms or palms.

There is an array of special devices known as assistive equipment that can offer help to those with osteoarthritis. Examples include elastic shoe laces, levers to turn faucets, handles that are built up to be thicker to be easier to hold forcefully. Also, a raised toilet seat, an extended shoehorn, tub grab bars and a shower seat offer protection for people with hip and knee problems.

*Surgery*     After all conservative treatments have failed to alleviate the pain and stop the advancement of osteoarthritis, a decision may be made to replace joints through surgery. By that time, the joint is virtually destroyed and the patient is usually suffering from severe pain. For many osteoarthritis patients, joint replacement is a wondrous cure that rescues them from being crippled or wheelchair-bound by the disease. Still, the decision to have joint replacement is considered to be an elective one since such surgery is not essential to preserve a patient's life.

Joint replacement surgery, a procedure that can restore function to almost any joint in the body, was pioneered in the late 1960s. Today, more than two million Americans have artificial joints. These devices are usually made of various metals and polyethylene, a plastic-like material. Often the implants are custom-designed for a patient by computer. An artificial joint consists of two parts. One part is a metal shaft that has a ball on the tip, which is wedged into a bone. The other part is a cup-shaped metal socket that has a plastic lining; this part fits into the adjacent bone. The ball then fits into the socket and swivels, allowing generous freedom of movement.

A decision to have joint replacement surgery is usually made when the pain of advanced osteoarthritis is so severe that it's hard to sleep at night or when normal activities have become greatly limited during the day. Your doctor will offer an opinion about undergoing the surgery based on the extent of the pain and disability, the condition of the bones and the strength of ligaments supporting the joint, as well as your overall health, including weight and physical condition and your own attitude towards the surgery. Although joint replacement is performed upwards of three hundred thousand times a year in the U.S., and with a high rate of success, there are risks associated with this surgery. Infection can occur, although it happens in only about one half a percent of cases. It is also possible that the artificial joint can become loose or dislocated.

Other surgical procedures such as osteotomy and arthrodesis, that were traditionally used to correct joints damaged by osteoarthritis, are not commonly utilized today because of the successful development of joint replacement.

Osteotomy is a procedure during which a wedge of bone is either removed or added, resulting in a realignment of a joint by shifting the weight bearing from one part of the joint to another. Arthrodesis is a method of eliminating pain and achieving stability by fusing two or more bones in a joint; it is used mostly for wrists. This procedure is a debilitating one, since a fused joint will lose its function.

Surgery on a much smaller scale is possible through use of the arthroscope, a small fiber-optic instrument that is commonly used in both diagnostic procedures and surgery. The arthroscope can be used to remove the so-called osteoarthritic debris, consisting of floating pieces of cartilage and bone fragments from the cavity of the joint.

## Alternative Treatments

The utilization of alternative therapies to cope with a chronic condition like osteoarthritis is widespread because the chance to obtain relief from pain without troublesome side effects is very appealing. Since the philosophy of natural remedies is one that places the nexus of managing pain within the province of the body itself, more and more arthritis patients have been turning to alternative treatments.

At the same time, the pain and disability of a long-term condition like osteoarthritis can lead people to such despair that they are susceptible to deceptive practices and unscrupulous sales pitches for nonexistent magical cures. More than two billion dollars are spent on unproven arthritis remedies every year by older Americans, according to the Arthritis Foundation. Many of those remedies not only are simply useless but are also dangerous and ought to be avoided. Typically, these are remedies that promise outright cures, immediate results or the capability to treat multiple disorders. Often these remedies are sold through mail order; a post office address is provided; and benefits are proclaimed through the testimonials of "cured" individuals.

However, this should not discourage you from considering the many natural treatments. They have been widely demonstrated to be effective and safe, although they have never been put to the scientific scrutiny that allopathic remedies routinely undergo. However, the Office of Alternative Medicine, created by the National Institutes of Health in 1992, has been conducting clinical trials on a number of alternative treatments which eventually may be helpful to people in their evaluation of possible treatments. Meanwhile, learning as much as possible about viable therapies and discussing the possibilities with your doctor are important procedures to undertake as a safeguard in avoiding harmful choices.

*Acupressure*   Pain can be soothed and mobility increased through acupressure treatments directed at the pressure points that correspond to specific joint locations. The best technique, which can be learned and self-administered, uses consistent, light pressure. Benefits of acupressure include reduction of pain and lessening of muscle tension, both of which result in an overall feeling of relaxation.

For joint pain that is located anywhere on the body, press both of the St 36 points, which are located several inches below each kneecap, in the indentation at the front of the shinbone. Pressing these points for about one minute three times a day will help to relieve pain.

*Acupuncture*   The technique of acupuncture is thought to reduce pain by releasing natural painkillers called endorphins and enkephalins which act like morphine to deaden pain. Practitioners of acupuncture believe that arthritis is the result of a blockage at the joint by the body's vital force or essence. An acupuncturist will determine a specific course of treatment for you after asking a series of questions about your particular symptoms and overall state of health.

Despite its growing popularity, however, many doctors and scientists believe that there is no physiological basis for the success of acupuncture and that it is successful only through a placebo effect.

**Aromatherapy**   Massaging aromatic oils into sore joints is a soothing treatment for lessening the aches of osteoarthritis. One common mixture consists of six drops each of rosemary and chamomile essentials added to four ounces of a carrier oil such as sesame, almond or avocado. Also soothing is the addition of ten drops each of rosemary and chamomile to a warm bath.

**Ayurveda**   An ancient system of healing based on five thousand years of folk wisdom from India, ayurveda works from the basic principle that the human body is a moving stream of submolecular particles that can be arranged and rearranged at will. Disease is seen as a state in which the particles are out of the order in which they normally flow. To loosen stiff joints and relieve pain, the suggested ayurveda remedy is to gently rub sesame oil on the affected areas, followed by a hot shower about twenty or thirty minutes later. Additionally, it is considered therapeutic to add spicy herbs such as cayenne, cinnamon and dried ginger to foods.

**Biofeedback**   The techniques of biofeedback can be harnessed to combat the painful symptoms of osteoarthritis. Using biofeedback techniques, a person is able to control certain body functions, such as decreasing the heart rate or altering brain rhythms. By using the same techniques to concentrate on relaxing muscle groups and eliminating muscle tension you can reduce pain. It does, however, take some time and practice to learn biofeedback techniques before being able to utilize them successfully.

*Flotation tanks*   Relief from chronic pain, especially stiff and achy joints, can be found through the use of flotation tanks. Today's tanks are not the earlier coffinlike structures that were called sensory-deprivation or isolation tanks. The new models are user-friendly, some with such features as a Jacuzzi, an intercom and a video screen.

When you float in a tank, you are drifting in a warm, buoyant liquid inside a light-free, soundproof chamber. Scientists have found that a person floating free of light, sound and touch can achieve a profound relaxation that triggers the same positive physical and mental effects as those that occur during meditation, which can linger long after the float is over.

As an aid in pain management, flotation tanks offer several benefits. First, buoyancy reduces pressure on the body and eases pain. More importantly, floating has been found to trigger the production of endorphins, the body's natural painkillers. Finally, a big advantage of flotation is that it serves as a natural form of biofeedback. Patients are able to concentrate on their breathing, heart rate and muscle tension, by learning how to deeply relax and alter bodily functions at will.

*Flower therapy*   The premise of flower therapy rests on the belief that flowers and essences stimulate the brain to release neurochemicals that can alter emotions such as fear, anger and anxiety. The result of these neurochemicals is believed to be a strengthening of the body's innate ability to heal itself. These flower essences are sold in a highly concentrated form, usually taken in one-fourth of a glass of water. Osteoarthritis is viewed by essence therapists as a condition in which the entire system has become somewhat acidic, a condition that is thought by many practitioners to be the result of hidden, unexpressed anger. A combination of the essences of holly and grapevine are identified as being able to remedy the condition.

*Food therapy*   The reliance on food as an aid to treating osteoarthritis is a subject of much controversy. There is no conclusive scientific evidence that certain foods can play a pivotal role in battling osteoarthritis. Since the symptoms of arthritis can suddenly emerge and just as suddenly disappear without any outside intervention, a remission of symptoms that is coincidental with a certain regimen can lead to unfounded claims. Thus, there have been some extreme recommendations such as that sufferers consume only white meat, eat dried rattlesnake meat or consume frequent doses of vinegar and honey.

Still, there are a number of recommendations regarding the role of diet in the treatment of arthritis that have gained broad acceptance. Generally, these recommendations focus on good nutrition and the avoidance of foods that are thought likely to trigger symptoms. Some studies have shown that a vegetarian diet is very beneficial in reducing and sometimes eliminating arthritis pain. A diet that is low in fat and sugar is thought to be beneficial because an excess of fat and sugar inhibits the body's ability to accept vital minerals such as calcium, magnesium, phosphorus and manganese, which are vital to healthy bones. Also important are dark green vegetables, rich in chlorophyll, because the center molecule of chlorophyll is magnesium. Magnesium helps to remove impurities from the bloodstream.

There has been much written about the need for people with arthritis to avoid the so-called nightshade vegetables—green peppers, eggplant, tomatoes, white potatoes. This is based on the belief that they contain a toxin called sotanine that can interfere with enzymes in the muscles and cause pain. While there is no scientific evidence in support of this, avoiding the "nightshades" has brought positive results for some people.

**Herbal therapy**   There are a number of herbs that are believed to be beneficial in easing the discomfort of osteoarthritis. These include alfalfa leaves, black cohosh, celery seed, chaparral leaves, valerian root and yucca extract. Herbal teas that are commonly recommended include brigham tea, comfrey tea, devil's claw tea, and parsley tea.

**Homeopathy**   A course of homeopathic therapy is devised after a homeopathist has reviewed all of the emotional and physical aspects of an individual. It's quite possible that two people with the same illness can have the same symptoms but will be given different remedies. To gain optimum results from using homeopathy as a treatment for osteoarthritis, a patient should consult with a homeopath for optimum results.

A commonly recommended homeopathic treatment for achy muscles of arthritis that worsen with cold and in the morning is 30 c of cimicifuga. Also two very popular remedies in treating painful joints are arnica and rhus toxicodendron.

**Massage**   A soothing massage can help to ease the pain of osteoarthritis, but it must be done gently. Put a little vegetable oil or massage oil on the fingertips so that the fingers will move easily over the skin. Don't massage the affected joint directly but rather work around it, staying just above and below the area with your fingertips. Make small, gentle circles around the joint for about three or four minutes each day.

**Nutritional therapy**    The role of nutrition has been embraced by many as an effective method for the treatment of osteoarthritis. In addition to the specific foods listed above, a number of vitamins have been identified as being useful in the treatment of osteoarthritis.

Niacin, also known as vitamin $B_3$, is used to help reduce joint pain and improve mobility. Niacin does occurs in its pure form in foods, but only in small or moderate amounts. The best sources include liver, poultry, fish and peanuts. As a supplement, a common dosage is in the range of 500 mg twice a day up to 1,000 mg three times a day.

Vitamin $B_{12}$, known to help boost the energy level and activity of the nervous system, has been useful in treating symptoms of osteoarthritis. However, it is difficult to acquire $B_{12}$ through a regular diet, although such foods as meats, oily fish and milk products contain it. One study of arthritis patients showed that taking a combination of vitamin $B_{12}$ and vitamin $B_1$ resulted in greater effectiveness of NSAID painkilling drugs. Thus, it is possible that the dosage of painkilling drugs could be reduced by taking a combination of $B_{12}$ and $B_1$. A recommended dosage is 100 mg of $B_1$ daily and 1,000 mcg of $B_{12}$.

Dietary supplements recommended by nutritionists include: primrose or salmon oil capsules, two capsules, twice a day; superoxide dismutase; calcium plus magnesium, 2,000 mg daily; coenzyme Q10, 60 mg daily; garlic tablets, two capsules three times daily; kelp, eight tablets daily; multienzymes, with meals; niacin plus vitamin $B_6$, 100 mg, three times daily; vitamin B complex with $B_3$, $B_6$, PABA (para-aminohemzoic acid) and $B_5$, 100 mg, three times daily; vitamin $B_{12}$ and folic acid, lozenges daily; vitamin C plus bioflavonoids, 3,000 to 10,000 mg daily in divided doses.

*Physiatry*    A small medical subspecialty called physiatry consists of physicians who have training in physical medicine and rehabilitation, including five years of specialty training after medical school. As rehabilitation experts, they work with other health professionals to devise and manage a treatment plan for patients who must make adjustments in their lifestyles following an illness or in the wake of a long-term, chronic ailment. For an osteoarthritis patient, a treatment plan might include heat and massage treatments, posture therapy, self-relaxation training and labor-saving ways of organizing chores. An advantage of consulting a specialist in physiatry is that the orientation is focused entirely on diagnostic and rehabilitative strategies, so you are likely to have a single, highly knowledgeable source for a multitude of practical and useful techniques.

*Poultice*    The use of poultice can relieve the pain of stiff or swollen joints associated with osteoarthritis. One of the solutions often suggested is a solution of two cups of Epsom salts in a gallon of warm water, in which a towel is dipped and then placed on the affected joint. After fifteen or twenty minutes, the towel should be removed and castor oil gently massaged on the area.

*Relaxation therapy*    Helpful in the management of pain from osteoarthritis is relaxation therapy. Particularly effective is a stretch-based technique. For example, weave your fingers together and raise your hands over your head, palms down. Then, straighten your elbows and rotate the palms outward until you can feel resistance. After holding the position for ten seconds, quickly release and then let your arms rest at your sides for one minute.

***Thermal biofeedback***   A special form of biofeedback called thermal biofeedback was developed at the Menninger Clinic. It is based on the idea that stress causes a restriction of the blood flow to the hands and feet, which causes them to become colder than the rest of the body. By using thermal biofeedback, you can warm your hands, thereby eliminating the stress and achieving a state of relaxation. Warm hands lead to an increase in the blood flow and a lessening of the stress hormones, resulting in relaxation of the muscles.

Most people can learn to use thermal biofeedback in one session. You simply sit down comfortably and place a thermometer across the fingers of one hand that is resting on your leg, palm side up; your other hand is palm down. Then, touch your fingertips together so that the little finger of each hand is touching the index finger of the opposite hand. Next, roll your fingers together so that they wrap around the thermometer and then rest your hands in your lap. Focus on trying to feel the signs of any sensation in your fingers. Keep focused and soon you should feel a tingling or pulsing in the fingertips, a sign that the hands are warming. You can look occasionally at the thermometer with the intention to warm it, but don't consciously try to raise the temperature of your hands. Let that occur naturally. The goal is to continue your focus until the finger temperature rises to ninety-seven degrees and hold it there for approximately ten minutes. After a time, you should be able to do this successfully without needing to use a thermometer.

## Combined Treatments

For some people with osteoarthritis, management of the disease amounts to an occasional need to handle achy pain, stiff joints and sometimes swelling. Others, however, must face not only the management of frequent pain on a long-range basis but also the possibility of the degenerative disease eventually destroying an entire joint. Still others will fall somewhere in between.

One thing is sure, however. More and more people are living longer in the U.S., increasing the likelihood not only of their having visible symptoms of osteoarthritis, but also of there being a more severe progression of the disease. In fact, the population of people over sixty-five grew by 100 percent during the last thirty-five years, while the overall population increased just 45 percent. The most rapidly growing elderly age group is the "oldest old," those over eighty-five which grew by 275 percent.

With osteoarthritis affecting a larger and larger percentage of the population, there will be even more attention and increased efforts devoted to the prevention and treatment of this disease. This means that virtually everyone should try to learn the basics about osteoarthritis and to keep up with treatment advancements.

Right now, for example, researchers are at work trying to develop a drug that can prevent osteoarthritis before it starts, by protecting the cartilage from deteriorating. There is also a drug under development that could stimulate the growth of new cartilage. If successful, doctors in the future could insert a temporary joint replacement that would dissolve as new cartilage forms.

With new treatment choices emerging and continued refinements of existing therapies, it's likely that a typical program to manage osteoarthritis will consist of a combination of allopathic and alternative approaches. Since virtually every patient has a unique experience with osteoarthritis in terms of the form it takes and the therapies that are undertaken, each person needs to take full responsibility for a personalized treatment program.

## Table 2

## TREATMENTS FOR OSTEOARTHRITIS

| Traditional | Alternative |
| --- | --- |
| **Acetaminophens**<br>Tylenol | **Acupressure**<br>St 36 points |
| **Topical analgesics**<br>methyl salicyclate; capsaicin cream | **Acupuncture** |
| | **Aromatherapy**<br>rosemary, chamomile essentials |
| **Aspirin**<br>buffered; coated; timed-release | **Ayurveda**<br>sesame oil; spicy herbs |
| **Nonsteroidal anti-inflammatory drugs (NSAIDs)**<br>over-the-counter ibuprofen (Advil, Motrin, Nuprin) prescription NSAIDs | **Biofeedback**<br><br>**Flotation tanks**<br><br>**Flower therapy**<br>holly, vine |
| **Heat therapy**<br>hot bath; whirlpool; moist hot pack<br>diathermy; ultrasound | **Food therapy**<br>low-fat diet; green veggies |

*Table 2 (cont.)*

| Traditional | Alternative |
| --- | --- |
| **Cold treatments**<br>ice pack | **Herbal therapy**<br>chaparral; celery seed;<br>  yucca; black cohosh;<br>  valerian; comfrey, devil's<br>  claw tea |
| **Exercise**<br>swimming; walking;<br>  X-country skiing;<br>  stationary bicycling | |
| | **Homeopathy**<br>cimicifuga; arnica; rhus<br>  toxicodendron |
| **Corticosteroids**<br>injections | |
| | **Massage** |
| **Occupational therapy**<br>adaptive equipment;<br>  preserving energy | **Nutritional therapy**<br>dietary supplements |
| **Surgery**<br>joint replacement;<br>  osteotomy; arthrodesis;<br>  arthroscopic procedures | **Physiatry** |
| | **Poultice**<br>Epsom salts |
| | **Relaxation therapy**<br>stretch-based |
| | **Thermal biofeedback** |

# CHAPTER 4

---

# Rheumatoid Arthritis

Rheumatoid arthritis is probably the most serious of all the one hundred forms of arthritis. This particular type of arthritis is inflammatory, not degenerative, so the fact that you are over the age of sixty or that you're a marathon runner with temperamental knees does not make you more likely than anyone else to contract rheumatoid arthritis.

There are 2.5 million Americans afflicted with this chronic condition, which strikes women three times more often than men. Peak years for its onset, which often begin gradually with subtle symptoms, are between ages twenty and forty-five.

Rheumatoid arthritis first appears as an inflammation of the membrane that lines and lubricates a joint. The tissues there are normally smooth and shiny, but once inflamed, they thicken and become swollen and painful. Often, movement of the joint is limited. Later on, this spreads to other parts of the affected joint, causing considerable stiffness and pain.

Most commonly affected are the small joints in the hands and feet, particularly the knuckles and toes. Rheumatoid arthritis can invade virtually any joint, especially those in the hands, feet, wrists, elbows, ankles, hips and knees.

People with rheumatoid arthritis often have accompanying symptoms of general malaise, including a low grade fever, decreased appetite, listlessness, fatigue and aching muscles. These symptoms are related to the systemic nature of inflammation and its tendency to affect more than one part of the body. Some patients will experience inflammation in various organs of the body, including the heart, lungs and eyes in addition to the joints.

Inflammation, a normal response within our bodies to infections and injuries, is produced when our white cells battle the invasion of infection. Typically, after an infection retreats or a wound is healed, the signs of inflammation will subside. However, the role of inflammation in rheumatoid arthritis is quite different. There seems to be a failure of the autoimmune system, which begins to fight the body instead of protecting it. Why does this happen? Just what causes rheumatoid arthritis? Research scientists have been at work on that question since 1858, when Sir Archibald Garrod first began exploring the mysterious disease, and still no single cause has been identified. Some possibilities that have been explored include genetic linkage, viral or bacterial infection and emotional stress. Research has concluded that no matter what is the cause of rheumatoid arthritis, it is not contagious and therefore it is impossible to catch from another person.

Rheumatoid arthritis is unpredictable in its nature and various among individuals as to what symptoms appear, how often they appear and what joints and organs are affected. Although it is a chronic disease, symptoms can appear in fairly long, separate occurrences, alternating with periods of remission during which there is reduced or complete absence of pain and stiffness. For some people, only one to two joints are affected while for others the disease may become widespread. In some cases, the disease disappears on its own and doesn't return. For others, rheumatoid arthritis becomes an ongoing debility for the rest of their lives.

Most people first notice the signs of pain and stiffness in their hands. Swelling is usually not present until a few months later. In perhaps two-thirds of all cases, the symptoms appear in matching joints, for example, the left and right elbows or left and right wrists. Other people may first experience either stiffness or progressively severe swelling only, without any pain. For a very few people, rheumatoid arthritis begins with one or two tender and swollen joints in an asymmetrical pattern, with the joints affected on one side being different from those affected on the other, for example, a right wrist and a left elbow.

Other symptoms that may be manifested include the appearance of red, painless lumps on the skin, known as rheumatoid nodules, located in the areas of the elbows, ears, nose, knees, toes or the back of the scalp. Also, there may be episodes of chest pain, labored breathing, dry mouth or dry and painful eyes.

The progression of rheumatoid arthritis, if left untreated, could take one of several different courses. The disease may recede for a period of time after little or no medical treatment. This spontaneous remission occurs in approximately 20 percent of all cases. More than half of these patients will have a recurrence at some time in the future; about 5 to 10 percent of untreated patients will have a permanent remission from rheumatoid arthritis.

Other patients will alternate occasional flare-ups of the disease with periods of normal health. Many people will not require any medications—for instance, if there is no evidence of damage to the joints and they remain fully functional. However, the attacks might appear frequently or last for long periods of time. Either situation could have an adverse effect, so that medication might be needed.

Another possible progression for a rheumatoid arthritis patient is recurring attacks without returning to a state of full wellness between them. In this scenario, there is a strong possibility of permanent damage to the joints because some inflammation is always present; medication should probably be considered.

Finally, another potential outcome is that the symptoms may increase in their severity slowly over time. Even though the progression of symptoms proceeds at a very slow pace, the result can be a rapid loss of joint abilities. Therefore, an early intervention with a treatment program to control symptoms is warranted to prevent permanent impairment.

Rheumatoid arthritis is a chronic condition for which there is no known cure. Statistics have shown that, in just under 50 percent of all cases, there is complete recovery of symptoms for a person after one or more episodes. Roughly the same percentage of people will remain somewhat arthritic. Perhaps 10 percent of those who have rheumatoid arthritis will have serious physical impairment from the condition.

The earlier that rheumatoid arthritis can be diagnosed, however, the more effectively it can be treated and with the most optimum results. The challenge is to have the presence of the disease clinically confirmed. Rheumatoid arthritis can be difficult to diagnose because it so often does begin very gradually with subtle symptoms. There are many other ailments that include pain in the joints as a symptom, so that a physician must explore a great number of other possibilities.

Added to those factors is the knowledge that this disease varies among individuals in its appearance and patterns. Even when a set of symptoms can be narrowed down to arthritis, remember that there are more than one hundred kinds of arthritis to consider, including other types of inflammatory arthritis, such as ankyslosing spondylitis, Reiter's syndrome, gout, systemic lupus erythematosus, psoriatic arthritis and arthritis-related colitis. Sometimes rheumatoid arthritis is mistaken for osteoarthritis, the most common type of arthritis.

If you have symptoms that suggest the existence of rheumatoid arthritis, the first step is to see your doctor. Take the time to think carefully about your symptoms beforehand, write them down and be ready to give as much detail as possible. The clinical history of your symptoms will be an important part of the data that a doctor will use in trying to make an accurate diagnosis. Information about your physical symptoms might include identifying all of the joints in which symptoms have occurred; indicating whether either pain, swelling or stiffness were present or a combination; establishing when the symptoms are at their most painful and what kind of treatment has diminished the pain.

In addition to the clinical history, a doctor will do a physical examination and perform diagnostic tests. Some tests are used to eliminate possibilities, while others are designed to confirm the presence of rheumatoid arthritis, to measure the level of complications and determine the effects of any medications.

The American College of Rheumatology recommends a number of criteria that could be relied upon to reach a precise diagnosis and arrive at the most appropriate treatment. These criteria for diagnosis of rheumatoid arthritis include:

the presence of arthritis for longer than six weeks; prolonged morning stiffness in the joints and muscles; presence of characteristic nodules under the skin; joint erosions apparent on an X ray; and positive blood tests for an antibody known as the rheumatoid factor.

Most likely, a doctor will utilize X rays, urine analyses, blood analyses and joint fluid analyses in carrying out various diagnostic tests. During the very early stages of rheumatoid arthritis, diagnostic tests probably will not actually confirm its presence, but they can be used to eliminate other conditions whose symptoms are similar to those of rheumatoid arthritis. There are a number of tests that are commonly used.

The rheumatoid factor test looks for an antibody called rheumatoid factor, or rheumatoid titer, which is present in the blood of close to 90 percent of patients who have rheumatoid arthritis. This test usually can be relied on to confirm a diagnosis of rheumatoid arthritis but it should not be used to positively exclude the possibility.

An erythrocyte sedimentation rate (ESR) test is used to measure the rate at which red blood cells settle or produce sedimentation. When inflammation is present, the red cells settle faster. The presence of inflammation doesn't confirm the existence of rheumatoid arthritis, however, since other conditions, such as infections, also produce high levels of inflammation. When used as a monitoring tool, this test can show changes in the level of inflammation, which is useful in evaluating the effectiveness of a medication in reducing inflammation.

Joint fluid analysis can be helpful as a way of confirming rheumatoid arthritis and excluding other types of inflammatory arthritis, as well as determining the presence of infection in the joint. Fluid from a joint that is exhibiting possible symptoms of rheumatoid arthritis is removed with a needle. If a sizable quantity of white blood cells called neutrophils are found, this can be a substantiating factor to confirm rheumatoid arthritis. The presence of infection can also be confirmed through analysis of the joint fluid. This test is also useful in eliminating other possibilities for the joint swelling. For example, if the fluid does not contain crystals, a number of other suspected maladies such as gout, bursitis and tendinitis can be ruled out.

A biopsy of the synovium, the lining of the joint, might be necessary when there has been no success in determining the cause of the patient's symptoms. This kind of test requires the withdrawal of tissue from the joint, using either a special needle or, more likely, an arthroscope. A skilled surgeon or other specialist is the best qualified to perform this procedure, which does involve a certain amount of discomfort. Analysis of the tissue can determine the presence of rheumatoid arthritis and exclude other possibilities.

X-ray studies of joints with symptoms of rheumatoid arthritis may not reveal any abnormalities during the early stages of the disease, even if a person is exhibiting fairly pronounced symptoms. However, X rays are useful in ruling out other causes of joint paint, such as fractures, bone infections or calcium deposits. During the course of the disease, a doctor will look for any signs of a thinning of the bone, indications of any small holes in the bone and any loss of cartilage from the joint. In some situations, more sophisticated kinds of imaging tests, such as magnetic resonance imaging (MRI), computed tomography scan ("CAT" scan) or bone scan testing, might be undertaken.

A number of blood tests have been used by research scientists at work looking for the cause of rheumatoid arthritis. They have isolated a genetic marker, HLA-DR4, on the surface of white blood cells that is present in 65 percent of rheumatoid patients. Since 25 percent of people without rheumatoid arthritis also have HLA-DR4, a genetic marker test would not be conclusive. It is thought, though, that the presence of these genes might indicate a person's susceptibility to developing rheumatoid arthritis.

Right now, the test is used only by doctors who work in research settings or at university centers. Another genetic marker, HLA-B27, is found in people who have other forms of inflammatory arthritis, notably spondylitis, which affects mostly the spine, as well as tendons and ligaments. This marker is also present in about 5 percent of people who do not have spondylarthropathy, so it's best used as a way to rule out other forms of arthritis when testing for rheumatoid arthritis.

Since diagnosing rheumatoid arthritis is a very challenging proposition in the earliest stages, there may be a matter of weeks or even months when there is a "wait and see" attitude. During this period, it's very important to keep an accurate record of any symptoms that occur and to follow all initial treatment strategies carefully so that you can assist your doctor in evaluating your condition.

## Traditional Treatments

Rheumatoid arthritis can be a mysterious and frustrating disease, with the prospects for a patient ranging from an improvement in the condition or a disappearance of the disease altogether to a situation where it might not get any worse or where it might progress into an increasingly more debilitating situation.

There has been a great deal of progress made in treatments and therapies for rheumatoid arthritis over the past forty years, however, allowing most people with this disease to attain good to excellent relief from their symptoms and to continue functioning at near-normal levels.

However, the characteristics and possible lingering effects of rheumatoid arthritis are far-reaching and therefore may require several types of treatment, including anti-inflammatory and pain medications, rehabilitation therapy, emotional counseling, and education in a number of areas such as exercise programs, joint protection, assistive devices and energy conversation.

Also, there are newer surgical treatments for rheumatoid arthritis that can provide significant benefits for many individuals.

A long-term care program should be undertaken as soon as possible, in order to maintain optimum function. There are two basic objectives in a treatment program: to relieve joint pain and to slow down the progression of the underlying disease. Your program most likely will be under the direction of a rheumatologist, a physician who is qualified by additional training and experience in the diagnosis and the treatment of various forms of arthritis. An experienced rheumatologist is familiar with the complex nature of rheumatoid arthritis and the many challenges involved in its treatment.

Medication is usually an essential component of any treatment program for rheumatoid arthritis. For many years, the traditional approach to medications has been to start during the first stage of the disease with the most conservative and safest types of drugs available, moving up to more powerful medications only when there was evidence that the disease had advanced into a more damaging phase.

In recent years, however, it has been determined that irreversible damage can occur during the early years, before it can be seen on X rays or in a physical examination. Today, therefore, many specialists believe that if a more powerful medication is used early on, there is a better chance of avoiding permanent damage. Some physicians even recommend a very aggressive treatment using several strong drugs, known as combination therapy, as early as within a few weeks of diagnosis. Meanwhile, research is ongoing in pharmaceutical therapy for rheumatoid arthritis treatments, and patients need to keep up with new developments and the latest recommendations in the field.

*Aspirin*     The single most widely used medication by rheumatoid arthritis sufferers is probably aspirin, despite the availability of many other prescription and nonprescription drugs. It is used not only to decrease inflammation but also to reduce pain and fever. However, the use of aspirin as an anti-inflammatory agent is effective only when it is taken in fairly large doses—on the average of from ten to twenty tablets a day. Unfortunately, at that level the chance of having harmful and unpleasant side effects is great.

The most common side effect is some form of stomach irritation such as nausea, indigestion or heartburn. More serious effects can include gastritis, stomach ulcers, bleeding ulcers, ringing in the ears and abnormal liver tests. Your doctor may want to experiment with various dosages and forms of aspirin, such as buffered, film-coated, enteric-coated and timed-release.

*Nonsteroidal anti-inflammatory drugs (NSAIDs)* A method of decreasing inflammation, pain and swelling that is just as effective as high doses of aspirin, nonsteroidal anti-inflammatory drugs (NSAIDs) generally result in fewer stomach problems. However, NSAIDs can produce a number of serious side effects, including upset stomach, heartburn, nausea, diarrhea, rash, weight gain, headache, drowsiness, dizziness, increased bleeding, ear ringing, stomach ulcers, gastritis, bleeding ulcers, kidney problems and blood problems.

Common NSAIDs include diclofenac, diflunisal, etodolac, fenoprofen, flurbiprofen, ibuprofen, indomethacin, ketoprofen, magnesium choline trisalicylate, meclofenamate, nabumetone, naproxen, phenylbutazone, piroxicam, salsalate, sulindac and tolmetin.

*Stomach medications* Often it is necessary to use medications to treat stomach problems that are created through the use of NSAIDs. These medications decrease the production of stomach acids, neutralize stomach acids or coat the lining of the stomach. Both prescription and over-the-counter stomach medications are commonly recommended for use. Misoprostol is commonly used to prevent stomach problems, but can cause cramping and diarrhea. Commonly utilized to decrease acid production are cimetidine, famotidine, nizatidine, ranitidine and prilosec. Sucralfate is used to coat the stomach. Over-the-counter antacids that neutralize acids include Maalox, Mylanta, Rolaids and Tums.

*Disease-modifying antirheumatic drugs (DMARDs)* It is possible to slow down the progress of rheumatoid arthritis and prevent joint damage through the use of disease-modifying antirheumatic drugs (DMARDs). In some instances, they may help to bring about complete remission of the disease. These drugs are also called slow-acting antirheumatic drugs (SAARDs) because they usually take weeks or even months to begin to work. Most common of the DMARDs are injectable gold, oral gold, hydroxychloroquine, penicillamine and sulfasalazine. Since they are slow working and have little effect in reducing pain, they are often taken in combination with NSAIDs. Doctors do not fully understand how and why these disease modifiers work, but they are very powerful and can produce serious side effects. Therefore, it is essential that your doctor maintain careful monitoring of your condition.

*Immunosuppressants* The use of immunosuppressants to decrease the hyperactivity of the immune system, which tends to be overactive in patients with rheumatoid arthritis, can slow down inflammation in joints. However, because the immune system is suppressed, the patient will have more difficulty fighting off infection. This, along with their side effects, means these drugs have the potential of being very dangerous. Possible side effects include nausea, vomiting, rashes and mouth sores, which usually can be controlled by changing the amount and frequency of the drug. More serious side effects include low white or red blood cell counts, liver damage, bleeding, bladder irritation and possible linkage to some forms of cancer. Common immunosuppressants are methotrexate and azathioprine. Any use of immunosuppressant drugs should be carefully monitored by your doctor.

*Corticosteroids* When a joint suddenly becomes very inflamed and painful, corticosteroids, which are very powerful anti-inflammatory drugs, may be prescribed for a limited time to help control disease flare-ups. While waiting for the slower-acting DMARDs to show results, corticosteroids may be substituted on a temporary basis for NSAIDs that have not produced results or have caused serious side effects. Many years ago, corticosteroids were used for long-term therapy and in high doses, but they caused such serious side effects that for many years their usage was eliminated entirely. Today, physicians prescribe them only in the smallest dosage possible, for the shortest length of time and only for patients who cannot take NSAIDs and DMARDs or whose rheumatoid arthritis is not being controlled successfully by a treatment program of NSAIDs and DMARDs. Corticosteroids need to be discontinued slowly and not abruptly—in fact, on a tapering-off schedule under your doctor's supervision.

Oral corticosteroids include betamethasone, cortisone, dexamethasone, methylprednisolone, prednisolone, prednisone and triamcinolone. Side effects include those that are immediate and those that result from long-term use. Most common of the immediate side effects are nausea, bloating and mood changes while cataracts, muscle weakness, susceptibility to infections and osteoporosis can result from long-term use.

Corticosteroid injections are used to treat a particular joint that has not responded to treatment as well as the other joints or a joint that has become more swollen than the others. A single injection will lessen the pain and swelling for up to six weeks. There are minimal side effects from corticosteroid injections, and if given not more than once every four months, there should be no adverse effects. Patients who have had corticosteroid injections need to avoid any activities that could put pressure on the joint, wear a splint for a wrist or possibly use crutches to prevent weight on a knee or ankle that has been injected. An ice pack, applied to the joint as soon after the injection as possible, will help to alleviate discomfort.

**Surgery**   One treatment option for patients with severe pain, limited movement and joint deformities is surgery. Through a variety of surgical procedures, severe pain can be controlled, inflamed tissue removed, ruptured ligaments or tendons repaired and joint function improved or restored.

A common surgical procedure used in the treatment of rheumatoid arthritis is a *synovectomy*, where the synovium, or joint lining, is removed. This is usually undertaken in order to prevent it from damaging other joint structures and cartilage. An open surgical synovectomy has been the surgical technique traditionally utilized but in recent years the arthroscope has been used as well. Arthroscopic synovectomy avoids cutting and opening the joint capsule surgically, as in open surgery, so recovery from this procedure is usually accomplished in very short time. Open surgery, however, does offer a better view and improved access into the total joint, so it's easier to accomplish a more thorough removal of the synovial tissue. New surgical techniques for removal of the synovium are being developed and include the use of laser, radiation and chemicals.

The arthroscope is still very useful in allowing a doctor the ability to see inside the joint without having the trauma of major surgery involved. As a diagnostic procedure, arthroscopic surgery helps a doctor analyze the conditions that are creating problems for the patient. It's also possible through use of the arthroscope to take a biopsy of tissue, repair ligaments and tendons and remove damaged cartilage.

*Arthrodesis* is a surgical procedure by which painful and unstable bones are fused together. Most often this is performed in the wrist, feet, ankles and thumbs. While it lessens pain and improves stability, motion is permanently restricted in the fused joint so it is not recommended for the hip or shoulder.

*Tendon transfer* is utilized in the repair of tendons and ligaments that have been damaged or ruptured by rheumatoid arthritis. This surgical procedure involves connecting an undamaged tendon to the ruptured one. This is used most frequently in the tendons that are located in the hand.

*Arthroplasty*, or joint replacement, was once reserved strictly for those older patients who were thought to be good risks for not wearing out new joints. Today, however, arthroplasty is having a major beneficial impact on people with rheumatoid arthritis. In recent years, there has been a shift in thinking among doctors, who now believe that being able to have functioning joints is a key element of wellness. The most common sites for joint replacement are the knees, hips and shoulders, while elbows, wrists and ankles are less frequent.

There are two methods used to attach artificial joints to the bone. In one approach, the stem of the replacement joint is inserted into a cement-filled hole that has been drilled in the bone. While there is a minimum of pain involved and a fast healing time associated with this method, there is the possibility that the cement will crack over time and the joint could loosen. In the second method, known as biologic fixation or cementless arthroplasty, the new joint contains a special porous surface. The new joint then is inserted into a hole in the bone, allowing the patient's own bone cells to grow into it and settle into place without the use of cement. The difficulties associated with this method are a longer healing time and rehabilitation, along with the possibility of there not being enough bone growth to support the joint with the desired stability.

*Exercise*　An important treatment strategy for rheumatoid arthritis patients is a carefully planned and managed exercise program, which can result in such benefits as easier movement, reduced pain and stiffness, higher self-esteem, a happier outlook, increased tolerance of pain and a more active social life. From a doctor's perspective, the goals of an exercise program for people with rheumatoid arthritis are to maintain range of motion, strengthen muscles, increase endurance, help joints work and move better, improve overall health and promote a sense of well-being.

An exercise program should be individually designed, taking into account the severity of the rheumatoid arthritis and the existing physical condition of the patient. Obviously, a person with very inflamed joints that are tender and swollen would not be a candidate for the same kind of exercise program that a person with stable joints and a minimum of stiffness and tenderness might be able to undertake. It is important to work closely with your doctor and, perhaps, a physical therapist, to design an exercise program that will be of optimum benefit. For rheumatoid arthritis patients, the best time to exercise is that time of day when they have the least pain and the most energy.

Range-of-motion exercises, in which each joint is moved as far as is comfortably possible in all directions, help to decrease stiffness and pain as well as to maintain flexibility and improve the functioning of the joints. Similarly, stretching exercises that stretch the joint just past a comfortable point also improve flexibility and the functioning of a joint. In combination, range-of-motion and stretching exercises provide an excellent warm-up before beginning an exercise program and are also useful at any time as a way to decrease stiffness in the joints.

Strengthening exercises increase the strength and tone of muscles, thus enabling the muscles to help protect the joints. Most doctors advise, however, that rheumatoid arthritis patients not exercise with weights to strengthen muscles because weight training can stress an inflamed joint. Additionally, any exercise that would involve moving the joints against high resistance should not be attempted. Instead, tightening the muscles through isometric exercises, by pushing or pulling against a fixed object without moving the joints, will promote muscle strength. For example, if you press on a wall without moving your shoulders, wrists or elbows but relying instead on the tightening or contracting of the muscles, you will strengthen the muscles while protecting the joints from stress.

A recent study by a team of doctors in the Netherlands has challenged the traditional viewpoint on the inadvisability of weight lifting for rheumatoid arthritis. In a group of one hundred arthritis patients, one group performed hour-long workouts three times a week that included intervals with hand weights and an exercise bike, while three other groups undertook various range-of-motion exercises. After three months, it was found that those who'd been exercising vigorously were not only in better shape altogether but had improved flexibility and muscle strength around their joints. While some patients did complain of joint pain during their workouts, it was with no more frequency than those who were only doing traditional stretching routines. As a result of this study, doctors in the future may look more closely at the content and level of vigor in the exercise programs that are recommended for rheumatoid arthritis patients.

Overall fitness and general health can be improved through endurance or aerobic exercises such as swimming, walking, bicycling and even some forms of low-impact aerobics, depending on the extent of arthritic involvement of lower extremity joints. Aerobic exercise improves your body's efficiency in using oxygen from the blood supply and also improves the circulation, respiration and functioning of the heart. Swimming is particularly recommended for rheumatoid arthritis patients because it offers most of the calisthenics inherent in land-based activities, while the buoyancy of the water supports your muscles and joints.

A good workout will include both strengthening and aerobic exercises as well as warm-up exercises and a cooldown. A cooldown period relaxes the muscles and wards off post-workout pain. Range-of-motion or aerobic exercises done in slow motion can be used as cooldown exercises.

***Occupational therapy*** A person's ability to perform daily tasks, adapt to disruptions in lifestyle and prevent loss of function can be aided by occupational therapy. Principles of energy conversion and joint protection, as well as techniques for stress management, are taught to minimize fatigue, reduce stress on joints, reduce pain and increase performance. Patients can learn alternative methods and the use of adaptive equipment for performing daily tasks for work, school, home and leisure in ways that take into account any physical limitations and also protect joints from added stress.

An underlying principle in planning and managing activities is to alternate those that require substantial energy with those that are less strenuous. This principle will help to preserve energy and also to protect joints. Splints worn around affected joints may be recommended to improve function, reduce inflammation, prevent contracture, provide stability and decrease pain.

It's a good idea to develop the habit of refraining from positions that promote misalignment or deformity of the joints. For example, when in the kitchen, stir with the thumb on top of the spoon as though holding an ice pick and make the circular motion with the shoulder instead of the hand. Refrain from leaning on your hands if you're standing against a railing. Try to avoid unnecessary wringing motions, instead letting washcloths dry or using an electric rather than a handheld can opener. Always use the largest joint and strongest muscle available. Therefore, try to open doors with power from the upper arm or even hip rather than from the fingers. When getting up from a sitting position, try to use the whole body to rise, avoiding pressure on the hip and knee joints. This involves sliding forward as far as possible, then leaning forward and swinging up, pushing off with forearms or palms.

There are an array of special devices known as assistive equipment that can offer help to those with rheumatoid arthritis. Examples include elastic shoe laces, levers to turn faucets, handles that are built up to be thicker. Also, a raised toilet seat, an extended shoe horn, tub grab bars and a shower seat offer protection for people with hip and knee problems.

***New treatments***  Since rheumatoid arthritis affects so many people, research into its cause and into developing treatments is ongoing and taking place on numerous fronts across many disciplines. Rheumatoid arthritis patients should keep abreast of new developments and discuss with their doctors if any of the new advancements would be beneficial.

For example, at the last annual meeting of the American College of Rheumatology, studies were released about a new therapy that utilizes a device called a PROSORBA column, a type of blood-cleansing device that works very much like a kidney dialysis machine. In this treatment, however, the device removed certain immune complexes thought to contribute to the inflammatory process of rheumatoid arthritis. After blood is drawn from the patient, plasma and cells are separated and the plasma is filtered through the PROSORBA column. The filtered plasma is remixed with the patient's own blood cells and is infused back into the body. A study of fifteen rheumatoid arthritis patients who received the treatment for twelve weeks resulted in significant reductions in pain and swelling—by as much as 76 percent—which still remained after six months.

## Alternative Treatments

Rheumatoid arthritis is a chronic disease that can have periods of spontaneous remission alternating with periods of brutal flare-ups. Day-to-day management of symptoms like stiffness, swelling and pain is therefore of primary concern. For a patient who is open and willing to try new approaches, there are dozens of alternative choices for treatment of rheumatic arthritis that promise relief from pain and without the sometimes severe side effects often associated with drug therapy.

Since the symptoms of rheumatoid arthritis can undergo spontaneous remission at unexpected times, a patient can never know with certainty if a particular treatment has truly engineered relief or not. And, since there is still so much that is not known about rheumatoid arthritis, including its cause and cure, there is little basis on which to dismiss alternative treatments summarily. At the same time, the painful, chronic nature of rheumatoid arthritis has inspired a number of unscrupulous promoters who prey on patients with absolute quackery.

Some of these treatments will not be harmful except as a waste of time and money, while others have the potential to cause a regression in health and well-being. Unfortunately, it's difficult to tell the potentially beneficial from the harmless and the harmful. But one sure sign of the unscrupulous is the promise of a cure, which should ring a warning bell to a patient. Other danger signs are treatments with extremely high price tags, an oral treatment without a list of ingredients given and a company with only a post office address.

*Acupressure*  Daily treatments of acupressure at the pressure points that correspond to specific joint locations can soothe the pain, reduce the inflammation and increase mobility. When the pressure points are lightly pressed, muscle tension relaxes and the muscle fibers lengthen, with the blood then flowing more freely to the joint, causing the swelling to reduce and the pain to disappear. In using acupressure on a chronic condition like rheumatoid arthritis, it's important to be persistent and consistent. For easing the pain of an acute flare-up, utilizing acupressure two or three times a day will produce optimum benefits. Later on, after relief is achieved, applying acupressure on a weekly basis can help to prevent recurrences.

There is one acupressure point that not only soothes discomfort in the neck but also lessens the overall irritability and discomfort of rheumatoid arthritis. Known as the "Gates of Consciousness" (GB20), the points are located below the base of the skull, about two inches out from the middle of the neck. Place your middle and index fingers under one side of the base of the skull, using the thumb of the same hand on the other side to press the GB20 points.

*Acupuncture*   According to acupuncture theory, the body's vital force or essence is blocked at the joints by one of the external factors of cold, damp, heat or wind, depending on the specific symptoms. An acupuncturist will ask a series of questions about your specific symptoms and then devise a course of treatment for you. Usually, acupuncture is very effective in treating rheumatoid arthritis, with the average length of a treatment program being about ten sessions. It is believed that acupuncture's success in reducing pain results from its ability to release certain natural painkillers called endorphins and enkephalins, substances that act like morphine to deaden pain. Still, there are plenty of doctors and scientists who believe that there is no physiological basis for its success and that it succeeds only through the placebo effect.

*Fish oil*   Special healing benefits have been linked to the omega-3 fatty acids that are contained in fish oil, which seem to aid in warding off heart attacks and lowering cholesterol levels. Now, recent studies indicate that fish oils can also benefit rheumatoid arthritis patients. A group of forty-six people undergoing long-term treatment in Australia consumed eighteen grams of fish oil daily for three months, with participants reporting fewer sore joints and increased grip strength. It is believed that the fatty acids work by suppressing the production of biochemicals that cause inflammation. For now, doctors believe that the best way to get fish oil is by eating fish, the ones most laden with omega-3, such as mackerel and bluefish. Fish oil supplements, doctors fear, can interfere too much with the ability of blood to clot and may even cause excessive bleeding. There is also believed to be a danger of it elevating levels of vitamin A and interacting poorly with other medications that are taken regularly.

*Flotation tanks*   For many patients, flotation tanks are a valuable source of relief from chronic pain, especially the pain of rheumatoid arthritis. Today's tanks are not the earlier coffinlike structures that were called sensory-deprivation or isolation tanks. The new models are user-friendly, some with such features as a Jacuzzi, intercom and video screen. When you float in a tank, you are drifting in warm, buoyant liquid inside a light-free soundproof chamber. Scientists have found that a person floating free of light, sound and touch can achieve a profound relaxation that triggers the same positive physical and mental effects as those that occur during meditation, which tend to linger long after the float is over.

As an aid in pain management, flotation tanks offer several benefits to rheumatoid arthritis patients. First, buoyancy reduces pressure on the body and eases pain. More importantly, floating triggers the production of endorphins, the body's natural painkillers. One study found that when people with rheumatoid arthritis floated twice a week, they remained pain-free for up to five days. Finally, a big advantage of flotation is that it serves as a natural form of feedback. Patients are able to concentrate on their breathing, heart rate and muscle tension, which is helpful in learning how to relax deeply and alter bodily functions at will.

***Food***    It is thought by many that food plays a major role in contributing to the development of symptoms of rheumatoid arthritis; this idea is based on the belief that food makes great demands on the immune system. Many foods contain allergens that the body must fight or adapt to by calling upon the immune system. The food allergies that are believed to aggravate symptoms of rheumatoid arthritis include wheat, corn, milk and other dairy products, eggs and beef. A study by doctors in England had twenty-two rheumatoid arthritis patients following a diet that was free of foods thought to be allergic. Twenty reported having their symptoms improve in approximately ten days.

People who have a more primitive diet, with a minimum of refined foods and foods with additives, are more likely to find relief from the symptoms of rheumatoid arthritis. Patients who eliminate sugar, saturated fat and refined carbohydrates and rely more on whole grains, fruits and vegetables have experienced great success in reducing painful symptoms; this is true especially among those patients who switched to a vegetarian diet.

While a number of nutritionally oriented doctors see great value in the role of diet for rheumatoid arthritis patients, however, it is a controversial subject; there are many in the medical profession who do not see any validity in that approach. In light of there being a fair amount of evidence that points to positive results from a modification of diet, it seems worthwhile for rheumatoid arthritis patients to try changes in their diet, especially since the recommended alterations in diet would at the very least contribute to a healthier pattern of eating.

***Herbal therapy***    The goal of herbal therapy is to remove toxic irritants and reduce the likelihood of an inflammatory response. In addition to having the patient remove sugar and animal fats from the diet, an herbal prescription might include celery seed (Apium graveolens), which stimulates the function of the kidneys, encourages digestive excretion and lowers levels of acidic waste products; wild yam (Dioscorea rillosa), which acts against inflammation and improves circulation to the extremities; dandelion root (Taraxacum officinale), a mild laxative and stimulant of the liver; and lignum vitae (Guaiacum officinale), which improves the blood supply to the extremities by widening the blood vessels and encouraging the cleansing of tissues.

*Homeopathy*  Homeopaths formulate their treatment based on all of the emotional and physical symptoms of an individual. So, depending on their emotional symptoms, a person who has a headache and a person with a rash might be given the identical remedy. At the same time, two people with the same illness can have different symptoms but will be given different remedies. Therefore, to gain optimum results from using homeopathy as a treatment for rheumatoid arthritis, a patient should consult with a homeopath.

Most commonly recommended homeopathic remedies for rheumatoid arthritis include bryonia, cimicifuga and rhus toxicodendron. Rhus toxicodendron is often used to relieve painful joints and stiffness located in the neck and small of the back, the kinds of joints that are worse in cold weather and feel better on warm dry days and after exercise. A typical dosage is 30 c daily or 12 c twice daily. The same dosage of bryonia relieves stiff and painful joints that are hot and swollen and that worsen with motion. And, for a general feeling of uneasiness, restlessness and achiness that worsens with cold and in the morning, 30 c of cimicifuga is considered to be an effective remedy.

*Hydrotherapy*    Depending on the kind of symptom and a patient's preference, hydrotherapy through the use of a moist heat pack or a cold wet compress for ten to twenty minutes every four hours will be soothing. A variation on the warm, moist treatment is to first rub eucalyptus-mint ointment on the joint and wrap the joint in plastic wrap before applying warm, damp towels. Most commonly, patients seem to prefer a warm compress for stiffness and dull, penetrating pain, and the cold compress for sharper, more intense pain. Also popular is a combination of hot and cold therapy through a contrast bath. In a contrast bath, the joint is soaked first in warm water for five minutes, followed by cold water for five minutes, finishing with five minutes of warm water.

*Imagery*    Strong concentration and a belief in the power of suggestion is necessary in using imagery. If you do the technique, you will first visualize the joint pain, giving it a shape, color and size. Concentrate on transforming it into a cloud and watch it float away, first out of your body, then out of your room, then out of the house and up into the sky. The technique should be used twice a day, ten to twenty minutes at a time.

*Juice therapy*    Some nutritionists urge the consumption of juices containing beta-carotene, as found in parsley, broccoli and spinach, and also juices with copper, found in carrots, apples and ginger. Pineapple juice is a source of bromelain, recommended because it has strong anti-inflammatory properties.

*Massage*    The swelling in rheumatoid arthritis is reduced when a gentle technique such as the effleurage stroke is used. It's important to use an oil or cream on the fingers to make the massage more gentle. Use long gliding strokes and gentle pressure to massage the muscle and tissue around the joint with your fingertips. Always stroke towards the heart and continue for five to ten minutes a day.

*Physiatry* A small medical subspecialty, physiatry consists of physicians who have training in physical medicine and rehabilitation, including five years of specialty training after medical school. As rehabilitation experts, they work with other health professionals to devise and manage a treatment plan. For a rheumatoid arthritis patient, a treatment plan might include heat and massage treatments, posture therapy, self-relaxation training, laborsaving ways of organizing chores. An advantage of consulting specialists in physiatry is that their orientation is focused entirely on diagnostic and rehabilitative strategies, so you are likely to have a single, highly knowledgeable source for a multitude of practical and useful techniques.

*Vitamin therapy* Rheumatoid arthritis patients can include various supplements in their treatment, with a number of different regimens recommended by nutritional specialists. Included in many formulations are borage oil, bromelain, copper, selenium, vitamin C, vitamin E, and zinc, as well as a multi-vitamin. You can devise an individualized combination based on your own dietary habits, research into the characteristics of various vitamins and consultation with a nutritionist.

*Yoga* A number of yoga hand exercises for rheumatoid arthritis can loosen the joints if done daily. In a typical exercise you begin by pressing your palms together in front of your body at stomach level. Then, open fingertips and palms, bending back at the wrists. Then bring your elbows together, moving your wrists away from each other and returning to the original position. Repeat this six times. Consult yoga books or classes for detailed information on various techniques.

## Combined Treatments

The traditional approach to rheumatoid arthritis, since it is a chronic disease with the cause and cure remaining unknown, is to focus on relieving the symptoms, with the hope of a spontaneous remission occurring. Since there is a great deal of pain associated with the symptoms, management of pain becomes an overriding focus for most rheumatoid arthritis patients. However, some of the most effective anti-inflammatory drugs have severe and alarming side effects.

A person with rheumatoid arthritis faces an enormous number of choices on how best to manage this complex disease. It takes a great deal of time to seek out and evaluate the therapeutic approaches that are available beyond conventional drug treatment. This is not a task to be undertaken alone. You need to work closely with your doctor and other medical practitioners. A patient must be willing also to experiment with various approaches and keep track of how each one meets expectations, fits into daily life and accomplishes the broader goals of the treatment program.

Be sure that you have one key medical professional who is knowledgeable and accepting of alternative approaches and how they might fit in with conventional treatment.

Combining conventional and alternative treatments is probably more the rule than the exception for rheumatoid arthritis patients because the relief of symptoms can best be accomplished through a multitude of techniques. Most physicians within the traditional medical community are familiar with the fact that there are many therapies that are successful even though they are not solidly grounded in scientific theory.

## Table 3

## TREATMENTS FOR RHEUMATOID ARTHRITIS

| Traditional | Alternative |
|---|---|
| **Aspirin**<br>buffered; coated; timed-release | **Acupressure** |
| | **Acupuncture** |
| **Nonsteroidal anti-inflammatory drugs (NSAIDs)**<br>ibuprofen, fenoprofen, flurbiprofen, etodolac, diflunisal, diclofenac, indomethacin, ketoprofen, magnesium choline trisalicylate, meclofenamate, nabumetone, naproxen, phenylbutazone, piroxicam, salsalate, sulindac, tolmetin | **Fish oil** |
| | **Flotation tank** |
| | **Food**<br>reduced fat;<br>vegetarian |
| | **Herbal therapy**<br>celery seed;<br>dandelion;<br>lignum vitae;<br>wild yam |
| **Stomach medications**<br>cimetidine, famotidine, nizatidine, sucralfate, prilosec, ranitidine, Maalox, Mylanta, Rolaids, Tums | |
| | **Homeopathy**<br>bryonia;<br>cimicifuga; rhus toxicodendron |
| **Disease-Modifying antirheumataic drugs (DMARDs)**<br>injectable gold, oral gold, hydroxycholoroquine, penicillamine, sulfasalazine | |

*Table 3 (cont.)*

| Traditional | Alternative |
|---|---|
| ***Immunosuppressants***<br>methotresafe; azathioprine | ***Hydrotherapy***<br>moist heat pack; cold wet compress; contrast bath |
| ***Corticosteroids***<br>betamethasone, cortisone, dexamethasone, methylprednisolone, prednisolone, prednisone, triamcinolone | ***Imagery***<br><br>***Juice therapy***<br>parsley, broccoli, spinach, carrot, apple, ginger |
| ***Surgery***<br>synovectomy, arthrodesis, tendon transfer, arthroplasty | |
| ***Exercise***<br>range-of-motion, stretching, strengthening, endurance, aerobic | ***Massage***<br>effleurage stroke<br><br>***Physiatry*** |
| ***Occupational therapy***<br>energy conservation; joint protection; stress management; adaptive equipment; assistive equipment; splinting | ***Vitamin therapy***<br>vitamin E, vitamin C, borage oil, zinc, copper, selenium, bromelain<br><br>***Yoga*** |

# CHAPTER 5

---

# Lyme Disease

Lyme disease is a systemic and infectious illness that is transmitted to humans by a tiny tick that is commonly known as the deer tick. The first noticeable symptom is usually a lesion at the site of a bite, along with fever, muscle and joint pain, headaches and other skin lesions. If not treated with antibiotics early, Lyme disease may progress to the heart, nervous system, joints and other organs.

There is probably no malady today that is more disconcerting to physicians, researchers and the general public alike than Lyme disease. There are forty distinguishable symptoms, which are liable to emerge over several stages, last many years and appear in various combinations that can easily be mistaken for any of nearly two hundred other ailments. No two people will have exactly the same symptoms.

Even the process for a laboratory confirmation of Lyme disease is by itself a daunting and painstaking ordeal, replete with tests that routinely and successively can register as false positive and false negative.

Finally, once clinically diagnosed with the condition, a Lyme disease patient can undergo weeks of treatment and be medically cured, yet continue to suffer from many of the symptoms for months.

The public awareness of some basic facts about Lyme disease, fanned by extensive and sometimes sensational media coverage, has resulted in the disease often being overdiagnosed. On the other hand, Lyme disease is sometimes underdiagnosed for people who are living in communities outside of the East Coast, the North Central states, and Northern California that have been identified as being high risk areas for contracting Lyme disease.

The adult deer tick that transmits Lyme disease is about the size of a poppy seed, perhaps one sixteenth of an inch across. Even smaller in size are the immature deer ticks, the nymphs, who are in a life-cycle stage just below that of the adult tick. It is the immature tick that is most active and most likely to bite humans and pass on the disease. Inside the gut of many, but not all, of the nymph ticks is a corkscrew-shaped organism called a spirochete, acquired when they bite and consume the blood of a white-footed field mouse in the Northeast or a wood rat on the West Coast.

Some of these infected ticks will go on to bite and infect previously uninfected mice. These mice can remain infected for long periods of time without any ill effects, while spreading the Lyme infection to the many ticks that then feed upon them. These ticks continue the cycle, spreading infection to other rodents and animals. Adult ticks prefer to feed on larger animals, especially deer, who are resistant to Lyme infection and do not participate in the cycle like the mice. However, the deer do provide blood nourishment for adult ticks and also carry them into areas where they did not exist before. Ticks also will travel to new geographic locations by attaching themselves to dogs, cats, rabbits, chipmunks, cattle, migrating birds, horses and other animals. As these animals continue to travel further, out of the known high-risk areas, so will the disease.

Lyme disease was named after the town of Old Lyme, Connecticut, where in 1975 there was a mysterious outbreak of what looked like juvenile rheumatoid arthritis, which affected thirty-nine children and twelve adults. After several years of investigation and research, the disease was traced to an ailment first described in Europe during the late 1800s and associated with a bite by a sheep tick. In 1992, the international medical community agreed to call the mysterious infection "Lyme disease" worldwide.

There are three areas of the country where the Lyme spirochetes, mice, deer and ticks are especially concentrated:

- The East Coast states of Massachusetts, Connecticut, Rhode Island, New York, New Jersey, Pennsylvania, Maryland and Delaware
- the North Central states of Wisconsin, Minnesota and Michigan
- Northern California

Infection of Lyme disease is most common during the summer months, when ticks are the most active and people are outdoors with their skin exposed. Note that any rash that occurs in the forty-eight hours immediately following a bite is due to an allergic reaction and is not Lyme disease. The first sign of Lyme disease in most patients is a small, slightly raised lesion at the site of the tick bite, surrounded by a red rash called erythema migrans, appearing at the site of the bite from three to thirty days after contact with the tick.

Later on, the rash may increase in size, and the central

portion will partially clear while the outer margins remain reddened, giving the rash a bull's-eye appearance. The rash can become quite large and may also be joined by one or more rashes emerging on other areas of the skin. The rash may be accompanied by a flu-like fever, chills, headache, sore throat, stiff neck, nausea, fatigue, inflammation of the eyes and vague aches and pains in muscles and joints.

Some people also will have swollen lymph glands. If there is a strong suspicion of Lyme disease at this early stage, based on known exposure to ticks and the observance of these symptoms, your physician might decide to begin a treatment that will prevent any further symptoms.

Unfortunately, symptoms of the early localized stage described above will appear in only 50 to 60 percent of Lyme disease patients. If you know that you've been bitten by a tick, but do not have the symptoms, there are several possible scenarios. One possibility is that the tick was not infected so you aren't either. The other possibility is that you were infected but just don't show any of the symptoms yet. And unfortunately, there is no test that confirms the presence of Lyme disease in the first stage. Only when the body begins to produce antibodies around four to six weeks after exposure, can testing have an opportunity to confirm a diagnosis.

When Lyme disease is not diagnosed or treated after the early localized stage, there are additional symptoms that can suddenly emerge as the bacteria begin to spread beyond the skin—a few weeks or many months later. As a systemic infection, Lyme disease that is unchecked can invade various organs progressively, including the heart, nervous system and other organs in addition to various joints. Symptoms of the second stage, called early-disseminated Lyme disease include new skin rashes that are much smaller than those in the early stage. About 50 to 80 percent of the people infected at this stage will develop arthritis in two or three joints. Perhaps 15 percent will have symptoms of the nervous system, including severe headaches, stiff neck, possible facial paralysis, sensitivity to bright light, tingling sensation in arms or legs, difficulty in concentrating, memory loss and changes in mood or sleep habits. About 8 percent will develop heart problems, such as palpitations, dizziness or mild shortness of breath.

These second-stage or early-disseminated Lyme disease symptoms can be displayed without a patient having any of the earlier symptoms and, on occasion, can occur in cases that had been treated in the initial stage. Since it may be months or even years after the actual tick bite that these symptoms present themselves, Lyme disease may not be suspected; the patient quite possibly never even saw the bite and/or never had symptoms. Instead, since these symptoms can suggest other diseases—such as multiple sclerosis, fibromyalgia, lupus, infectious mononucleosis, Lou Gehrig's disease (amyotrophic lateral sclerosis) and Alzheimer's disease—patients may be going from specialist to specialist trying to find a definitive diagnosis.

Late or chronic Lyme disease, which can begin as early as six months after the initial infection or sometimes not until several years later, is characterized by severe arthritis, generally in only one of the joints, usually the knee. There can also be continued problems of the nervous system, including loss of memory, tingling and numbness in the arms and legs and trouble concentrating. Even if the disease is finally diagnosed, treatment at this stage may not effectively end these symptoms, especially the chronic arthritis.

Obviously, this disease can be severe and devastating if treatment is not obtained. Ironically, the course of treatment is fairly uncomplicated; getting the confirmation of its existence is the challenge.

Ideally, confirmation of Lyme disease is best done at approximately six weeks after someone has been bitten by the tick, especially if there have not been any symptoms. This is because it takes from four to six weeks for the body to produce the antibodies against the Lyme infection that can be measured in a test.

Suppose you know that you have been bitten by a tick, should you wait for six weeks to begin testing or should you begin taking the antibodies immediately, just in case? The problem of taking antibiotics immediately on the chance that it might be Lyme disease is that the drugs will prevent any antibodies from forming, so the disease cannot be confirmed at six weeks. However, if the telltale symptoms begin to appear sometime after forty-eight hours, it's probably Lyme disease and treatment ought to be started. If no symptoms appear after six weeks, then it might be wise to have testing done.

The medical research community is continuing to look for new, improved testing for Lyme disease because there is as yet no single, totally dependable test that can be expected to produce conclusive results. That is why testing usually consists of more than one type. Patients are tested first with the ELISA (enzyme-linked immunosorbent assay), followed by the Western blot. If there is still ambiguity after those two tests, a patient should visit a Lyme disease specialist, preferably one who is affiliated with an academic medical center.

## Traditional Treatments

The good news about Lyme disease is that traditional antibiotic therapy is very effective in fighting it. The specific medication that is used will depend on the stage of the disease, the kinds of symptoms and their seriousness, age of the patient and any existing allergies.

About 15 percent of patients will experience an increase in symptoms, such as fever, redder rash and overall body discomforts, during the first day or two of antibiotic therapy. Called a Jarisch-Herxheimer reaction, there is no reason to be concerned; it is thought to be caused by the bacteria dying and releasing fluids that are irritating to the body. The Jarisch-Herxheimer reaction ends by itself after a day or two.

*Tetracycline*   A drug that is commonly recommended for treatment of Lyme disease in its early localized stage is tetracycline. If the patient is under eight or still has baby teeth, tetracycline should not be given because it will stain baby teeth. In such cases either amoxicillin or penicillin would be a better choice. Other choices of medication include cefuroxime axetil, doxycycline, or erythromycin.

*Amoxicillin*   A prolonged high dose of amoxicillin is a recommended antibiotic for treatment during the second, early disseminated stage of Lyme disease. Also frequently prescribed are tetracycline and doxycyline.

*Penicillin or ceftriaxone*   The common treatment for Lyme disease in its late/chronic stage is either penicillin or ceftriaxone, given in a high dosage intravenously.

*Over-the-counter pain relievers*   An effective way to reduce the pain and inflammation of Lyme disease is through the use of over-the-counter pain relievers.

## Alternative Treatments

The role of alternative therapies in the treatment of Lyme disease is for the most part complementary to the antibiotic medication that will have been prescribed already. The various treatments that are most widely utilized focus on helping to ameliorate some of the accompanying symptoms of Lyme disease, to strengthen the body's immune and energy systems and to work towards regaining an overall state of wellness.

*Acupressure*  The Lyme disease symptoms of both arthritic pain and migraine headaches can be treated through the techniques of acupressure. To relieve the discomfort of a headache, draw an imaginary line from the center of the forehead back to the base of the skull and apply pressure at each point along the way, utilizing the bulb of the thumb. Then, using both hands, press points from the crown of the head to the temples. Press points on each side of the head simultaneously, about an inch apart. In treating arthritic pain, locate the correct points, based on where the pain is and which acupressure points correspond.

*Acupuncture*  Patients who are recovering from Lyme disease can benefit from acupuncture. These treatments help to raise levels of general wellness and strength by realigning the various energy systems in the body as well as boosting the immune system. Additionally, the arthritic pain of specific joints can be relieved by utilizing the specific acupoints that relate to those joints.

*Aromatherapy*  A soothing technique to relieve the headache pain associated with Lyme disease is aromatherapy. One method is to add a drop of peppermint essential oil to a small amount of unscented facial lotion, then lightly smooth the lotion under the nose and behind the ears. Another method is to inhale the peppermint from the bottle.

***Chiropractic*** Regular chiropractic treatments can assist in strengthening the body's energy systems, which have been adversely affected by chemical stresses that have in turn resulted in symptoms of chronic fatigue. Through chiropractic adjustments, energy flow and circulation can be improved.

***Food therapy*** The most beneficial diet is one that is rich in garlic and foods containing vitamin C, which can lessen the flu-like effects of Lyme disease. All varieties of citrus fruits and strawberries, kiwi, melons, raspberries, peppers, tomatoes, spinach, cabbage and broccoli are among the foods rich in vitamin C. To help overcome memory problems, try consuming at least one serving of foods that are rich in beta-carotene, like dark green vegetables, orange fruits and orange vegetables.

***Herbal therapy*** A relaxing method of easing headache pain is by drinking a cup of herbal tea. Recommended is a tea brewed from a combination of equal parts of wintergreen, willow bark and meadowsweet. Pour boiling water over a teaspoon of the mixture and let it steep for ten minutes. After straining, cool the tea to a desirable temperature and drink it.

***Homeopathy*** The objective of a homeopathic treatment for Lyme disease is to draw the Lyme spirochete out of the body's cells and into the bloodstream, where the homeopathic substance can stimulate the body to take action against it. A homeopathic practitioner will consider the individual.

***Hydrotherapy*** Relief from the severe joint pain that is associated with Lyme disease can be obtained through hydrotherapy. For a dull, penetrating pain, try placing a warm compress directly on the affected area. Be sure that the compress is not too hot but is rather a temperature that is comfortable. An ice pack works best in treating a sharp, intense pain. Use an ice pack that is wrapped in a plastic bag and place it over a towel on the skin, holding it in place for approximately ten to twenty minutes. Repeat the hot or cold treatment every four hours until there is relief. To relieve a stiff neck, soak a towel in hot water, then wring it out and apply it to the back of the neck.

*Imagery*    A healing technique that many people may not be comfortable utilizing is imagery. The patient must have not only a strong belief that it can work but also the determination to continue utilizing the technique on a daily basis until it's successful.

As a Lyme disease patient, you need to be able to visualize the spirochete, the coiled-shaped organism that causes the disease, as a brown bug with a round body and eight legs. Then, envision several such bugs swimming in your bloodstream, while you swim nearby with a candle or a blowtorch. Point the candle or blowtorch at one of the spirochetes and watch it shrivel up. Keep doing this until all the spirochetes are dead. Then, visualize yourself in a recovering state. It is suggested that you repeat this once a day in the morning.

Imagery can also be used in treating headaches. Just imagine that all of the muscles in the neck and head are springs that are tightly coiled. Slowly, imagine that these springs are starting to become loose. The muscles should relax and the pain will begin to lessen.

***Kinesiology*** A multifaceted treatment system, kinesiology incorporates nutrition, exercise and acupressure. This focused approach can replenish and strengthen the body's weakened system. A practitioner of kinesiology might be an osteopath, a chiropractor or an allopathic doctor.

***Massage*** A stiff neck that is associated with Lyme disease can be treated effectively through massage. One form of massage that can be self-administered utilizes a standard bath towel. First, fold the towel lengthwise, bringing the sides to the middle until the edges touch, then roll up the towel snugly. Next, lie down flat on your back on either the floor or a mat and place the towel directly under the curve of your neck. Hold this position for fifteen or twenty minutes. Another exercise is to fold the bath towel lengthwise into thirds and hold onto one end in each hand. Place the middle of the towel behind your head at the base of the skull and then relax, letting your head fall back onto the support of the towel. Then, pull the towel back and forth with your hands, letting your head being pulled with the towel.

***Nutrition*** The aim of nutritional supplements is to strengthen the immune system. Recommended nutrients include: chlorophyll, taken daily; garlic capsules, two capsules three times daily; five tablets of kelp daily; 100 to 200 mg. of germanium daily; a high potency multivitamin daily; 200 mcg. of selenium daily; 50,000 IU of Vitamin A daily; 10,000 mg. of Vitamin C daily; 600 IU of Vitamin E daily.

***Physical therapy*** An ongoing program of physical therapy is recommended for Lyme patients as a way of helping them to regain strength and stamina. Patients are advised to begin physical activities such as swimming, aerobics, and walking at a slow pace, gradually building up the pace and length. Afterwards, it's a good idea to have a hot bath followed by a nap.

**Reflexology techniques**   The techniques of reflexology are often used to counteract the various flu-like symptoms of Lyme disease. Apply pressure to the hands and feet, working the reflex points for the chest and lung, diaphragm, intestine, lymphatic system and pituitary and adrenal glands.

**Support groups**   People who have long-term or ongoing diseases often form support groups, which provide both educational and emotional assistance. For people who have Lyme disease, there are many support groups, as well as foundations, newsletters, activist groups, research centers and educational organizations. Within support groups, patients can share experiences, gain additional knowledge and express their feelings. Having the emotional support and connection with people who are battling the same disease can be a powerful aid to healing.

## Combined Treatments

Once a prescribed treatment of antibiotics is underway, a Lyme disease patient can look to a variety of additional, alternative therapies that may help to relieve the numerous painful symptoms that are associated with the disease. Virtually every patient has a unique set of symptoms and will need to put together a personalized program of treatment. It's important to discuss with your primary physician whatever alternative, complementary treatments you are considering to be sure that the effectiveness of the antibiotic treatment will not be compromised in any way.

## Table 4

---

### TREATMENTS FOR LYME DISEASE

---

| Traditional | Alternative |
| --- | --- |
| *Medication* | *Acupressure* |
| tetracycline; amoxicillin; penicillin; doxycycline; cefuroxime axetil; erythromycin; oral dosage—early localized stage (antibiotics) | *Acupuncture* |
| | *Aromatherapy* |
| | peppermint oil |
| amoxicillin; tetracycline; doxycycline; prolonged high dosage orally—early disseminated stage (antibiotics) | *Chiropractic* |
| | *Food therapy* |
| | garlic, foods rich in vitamin C |
| penicillin; ceftriaxone; high dosage intravenously—late/chronic stage (antibiotics) | *Herbal therapy* |
| over-the-counter pain relievers | wintergreen; willow bark; meadowsweet |
| | *Homeopathy* |
| | *Hydrotherapy* |
| | heat, cold |
| | *Imagery* |
| | *Kinesiology* |
| | *Massage* |
| | *Nutrition* |
| | *Reflexology techniques* |
| | *Support groups* |

# CHAPTER 6

---

# Bursitis

Bursitis occurs when a bursa becomes inflamed or irritated. A small, fluid-filled sac located in or near a joint, the bursa functions as a cushion between the muscles, bones and tendons. There are at least one hundred fifty bursae located throughout the body. By producing a lubricating fluid, the bursae are able to minimize friction and help the joints move smoothly.

Whether it's in the dark chambers of dusty coal mines, the far-flung venues of the professional tennis tour or the well-scrubbed patio of a spacious vacation home, overdoing and overreaching at work, at home or at play can exact a toll on the body. Fanciful names like "miner's elbow," "tennis shoulder" and "housemaid's knee" are commonly used to describe forms of the same painful condition, which is called bursitis.

Trauma, strain, infection or arthritis can all lead to bursitis, but repetitive motion is the most common cause. The areas where bursitis is most likely to develop are the shoulder, hip, elbow, wrist, heels, knees and the base of the big toe. It is the inflammation of a tiny bursa in the big toe that actually causes the formation of a bunion. (see chapter 10, Bunions).

Movements that are repeated many times or in an awkward position, especially if the person has poor posture or is not physically fit, can cause inflammation of the bursae. For example, the tennis player who modifies the overhead motion of a serve, then practices it for prolonged periods of time without respite, could be a prime candidate for bursitis. Overuse of the hip muscles can create bursitis in the hip, called "snapping hip." Race walkers, female runners with a wide pelvis, cyclists, swimmers and players who take part in contact sports are commonly affected. The repetitive motion of swinging a pick all day long is what leads to miner's elbow. And at home, pushing a vacuum back and forth can also lead to an inflamed bursa.

Bursitis can also be the result of prolonged or excessive pressure. Housemaid's knee, for instance, is a soft, egg-shaped bump that forms on the front of the knee after long periods of kneeling on the floor while scrubbing it. Years ago, "weaver's bottom" was diagnosed among hardworking artisans who sat on a hard surface and worked for long hours at the loom, swaying back and forth during the process.

The first symptoms of bursitis are stiffness in the joint area and a pain that is aggravated by movement and that may be more prominent at night. There also may be some swelling in the joint area, and the surface of the skin, when touched, will feel as if there is fluid inside.

There are two phases to bursitis. The first phase is the acute stage, which can be very painful; during this time any movement of the affected area is liable to increase the inflammation. After the intensity of the pain lessens, usually after four or five days, there is a second phase lasting from approximately ten days to two weeks during which there is continued healing and rehabilitation.

There is a possibility that the joint pain is actually caused by arthritis and not bursitis, and therefore would require a long-term treatment program. An accurate diagnosis requires a review of your medical history and a physical examination. It may be necessary to have X rays, on which bursae are not visible, to exclude bony abnormalities or arthritis as the cause of the symptoms. When rheumatoid arthritis or diabetes is suspected as an underlying condition, blood tests may be recommended.

It is also possible that the problem is an infection or gout, which can be tested by aspiration of the bursa. Bursitis caused by an infection is called septic bursitis, an condition that is liable to spread or become severe. When that occurs, drainage of the bursa may be necessary. However, when it is properly diagnosed at an early stage, septic arthritis responds well to antibiotics.

Once diagnosed, most bouts of bursitis do not require a physician's help, although persistent pain that does not follow the normal course of bursitis should be investigated by your doctor. Most instances of bursitis will subside completely within two weeks, but there is a tendency for the condition to recur in many people.

There are a number of commonsense techniques that can help to prevent bursitis from recurring:

- Always wear protective gear when playing sports. Make sure that you're using the proper techniques for a particular sport, as awkward or incorrect posture can be harmful.
- Don't overdo repetitive physical activities; avoid extremely strenuous tasks.

- Whenever you must work in a kneeling position, be sure to use knee pads or cushions, take regular breaks by standing up for a few moments, and change positions frequently.
- Wear high heels as little as possible, and be sure to replace running shoes when they wear out.

## Traditional Treatment

Although bursitis is not a serious medical problem, it is a very painful condition that, if not treated properly, can result in permanently incapacities. This means it is of utmost importance to keep in mind and adhere to the two distinctly different treatment approaches for the early, or acute, stage and the second stage of the condition.

During the acute stage, cold packs and immobilization of the joint area are needed, while in the second stage, applications of heat are recommended. Also, it is extremely important that proper exercise of the area be undertaken once the critical stage is over. Otherwise, there is a chance that crippling adhesions will develop and that the joint will eventually "freeze up."

**RICE**   The key elements of initial treatment for bursitis are rest, ice, compression and elevation (RICE). This treatment is very helpful during the first five days and especially on the first day, for limiting the immediate pain and inflammation. During this time, you can use the RICE technique nonstop for the first few hours, then gradually decrease it to perhaps a half dozen times on the second day, less frequently on the third.

Resting the injured part by immobilizing it will help to avoid further inflammation, and it minimizes the pain. Limit your movement to the very minimum. A sling can be used to immobilize a shoulder or elbow.

Ice applied to the injured joint as soon as possible is the most beneficial of the RICE components because it reduces swelling and inflammation. It's important to reduce swelling because swelling can damage cells by decreasing oxygen to the surrounding tissue. Application of cold slows down metabolism within the cell and allows tissues to survive the temporary lack of oxygen. This procedure speeds healing by promoting the renewal of cells. Cold also helps to relieve pain by numbing the area and preventing nerves from sending pain messages to the brain.

The ice can be applied in a number of ways. However, it's important that ice not be placed directly on the skin because that can cause frostbite or tissue damage. A bag of frozen vegetables from the freezer can function as an instant ice pack. Or, put some crushed ice in a plastic bag and wrap it in a towel or cloth. There are also instant, disposable cold packs that are chemically activated and last for about twenty minutes; reusable cold packs are first cooled in the freezer.

Apply ice to the area for no more than twenty minutes at a time because there's always a possibility of frostbite. It's all right for the area to be reddish and slightly numb, but if it turns white or blue, stop treatment immediately. And if you have a vascular disease, rheumatism or decreased sensation, speak to your doctor before applying ice.

Compression helps to limit bleeding and reduce the swelling. Wrap the joint with strips of cloth in a figure-eight pattern, an Ace-brand bandage or other kind of elastic bandage. Don't wrap the area too tightly, or the circulation may be cut off. The fit should be firmly snug but not tight. Check periodically for signs of inadequate circulation such as tingling, numbness, loss of motion or blue skin. One good method is to have the ice and compression on for twenty minutes, then remove them for fifteen minutes.

Elevation of the injured area above the level of your heart will help to drain blood and fluids from the joint and to reduce swelling.

***Over-the-counter pain relievers***   Effective agents to reduce pain by lessening the inflammation are over-the-counter drugs such as aspirin and ibuprofen (Advil and Nuprin). However, be careful to watch the dosage and do not exceed it; an excess amount can cause stomach irritation. Do not take any of the acetaminophen products (e.g., Tylenol) for bursitis, because they do not contain anti-inflammatory ingredients.

***Nonsteroidal anti-inflammatory drugs (NSAIDs)***   In some instances, it may be appropriate to prescribe NSAIDs, or nonsteroidal anti-inflammatory drugs, to reduce the swelling and to relieve pain and stiffness.

***Corticosteroids***   It may be necessary to inject a corticosteroid into the affected area, along with a local anesthetic, to relieve pain and to educe inflammation.

***Fluid withdrawal***   Your doctor may recommend withdrawing fluid from the bursa by using a needle to syringe it.

***Surgery***   Removal of the bursa through surgery is rarely performed but may be warranted in severe, persistent cases.

***Heat treatments***   The application of heat after the inflammation has subsided will continue to aid the healing process. The general rule is not to begin to apply heat until the area is no longer hot to the touch. A heating pad or a warm, moist cloth is effective. It's especially beneficial to undergo heat treatment just before an exercise period, because the heat will draw blood to the area, reducing pain and permitting freer motion of the joint.

*Ultrasound therapy*  A safe and effective method to alleviate bursitis is through ultrasound therapy, the use of high frequency sound waves. The sound waves heat injured tissue and increase the blood circulation.

*Exercise*  As soon as the acute pain and swelling have receded, exercise of the joint should be commenced. Exercise will help prevent atrophy and stiffness, and it aids in achieving full movement and use of the joint eventually. This process should be approached slowly and carefully, however, and the exercise should last only a minute or two at the beginning, to be repeated again during the day. Care should be taken to support the injured area, especially for the first several days. For example, an arm should be allowed to swing in every direction, gently, but supported by the other arm.

Remember that the objective is not to build the muscle strength but to attain mobility and increase the range of motion. All that is needed and recommended is to gently move the injured part in ever larger circles for a few minutes, several times throughout the day. Keep doing the exercise each day, increasing the duration and intensity until the joint can move freely and fully. It's important to stick with this routine because a joint left unused might develop adhesions, then freeze up, leaving a permanently immobile condition.

Once there is no more pain and the range of movement is back to normal, you can resume regular exercise. In some cases, however, a joint will not move easily and a doctor is needed to help restore movement to the joint by manipulating it for you at the beginning.

## Alternative Treatments

*Acupuncture*   Since acupuncture is a widely used method of coping with all forms of arthritis, it has become a popular method of alternative treatment for bursitis, which is classified as a form of nonarticular arthritis.

*Castor oil heat treatment*   To soothe and continue the healing of bursitis, spread castor oil over the area of the affected joint and cover with cotton or wool flannel; then apply a heating pad.

*Contrast treatments*   Once the initial, acute pain has subsided, the use of alternating applications of heat and cold is a way to continue reducing the pain and swelling. A good method is to apply an ice pack for fifteen minutes, followed by a warm compress for fifteen minutes, then back to the ice, and so on.

*Food therapy*   There are several foods that are thought to aid in the recovery process by reducing the inflammation of the bursa. In particular, barley green is recommended; available in most health food stores, it can be sprinkled on a salad. Also, the consumption of pineapple is helpful because it contains bromelain, a natural anti-inflammatory ingredient.

*Homeopathy*   The use of homeopathy in treating bursitis can be either by injection or as an oral remedy. Ruta grav is the remedy that is most often injected. Popular oral remedies, consisting of four pills four times a day until better, include: ruta grav, especially when soreness and stiffness get worse after prolonged motion; rhus toxicodendron, if the joint is very stiff and feels better after continued motion; benzoic acid, when the joint cracks after motion and there are painful nodules; bryonia, if the area is red hot and swollen and it feels worse with any motion. After initial treatment with any of these oral remedies, follow with a single dose of Calcarea fluorica.

*Herbal tea*   A soothing technique for easing the pain associated with bursitis is the consumption of herbal tea, particularly at bedtime. Often a strongly brewed cup of chamomile alone can be sufficient. A more potent tea, consisting of two parts chamomile, one part lady's slipper and one part skullcap, is quite effective. At bedtime, hops and passion flower added to the mixture will help bring about a more restful sleep.

*Massage therapy*   The pain and stiffness of bursitis can be eased through massage therapy, as long as gentle stroking is used. Don't massage the joint directly, because that could create additional pain and inflammation. Instead, concentrate on the thickest part of the muscle near the joint. It's best to spread massage oil, scented oil or even vegetable oil on your hands. Begin by warming up the area by lightly stroking the area, using long gliding strokes and a soft pressure. Do this for several minutes. Then, use the fingertips and thumbs to make small, circular movements on the muscle. The fingertips remain stationary and work through the skin to the muscle below. Vary the pressure, starting with a very light touch and increasing it slightly after a minute or two. For a large area, you can use the palm or heel of the hand.

*Nutrition therapy*   The role of nutrition in lessening the effects of bursitis has been recently recognized. Of particular importance in overcoming acute inflammation is an enzyme that is combined with several antioxidants. Although routinely used as a digestive aid, Inflazyme Forte can be a powerful aid in reducing acute inflammation. Suggested dosage is two tablets between meals.

Another valuable nutritional aid in healing bursitis is a combination of calcium and magnesium, which together help to build and strengthen bones, in a daily dosage of 1,500 mg of calcium and 750 mg of magnesium.

Additionally, vitamin C, which promotes the growth and repair of cells, should be taken in large doses during the healing period—some people suggest as high as a total of 3,000 to 8,000 mg daily.

Vitamin A reduces inflammation and aids in the repair of tissues. During the acute phase and for perhaps a month, 100,000 IU daily, then reduce the dosage to 50,000 IU daily, and after two more weeks, down to 25,000 IU daily.

Vitamin E also works to reduce inflammation and encourage healing, starting with a dosage of 400 IU daily, increasing to 1,000 IU over time.

*Poultices*    Composed of herbs or other natural substances that are mashed together and then heated, poultices can soothe sore areas, speed healing and purify the area by drawing out foreign matter. However, since they are messy and labor-intensive to prepare, poultices are not in common usage.

Among the best is the comfrey poultice, prepared from either the fresh leaves, dried leaves or chopped roots of comfrey. Put the comfrey in a pan and cover with water, then bring to a boil. Once the water begins to boil, remove the pan immediately from the stove and let the mash cool until is warm but not uncomfortably hot. Spoon the mash between layers of gauze and apply to the injured area. If any minor irritation occurs, rub lanolin or olive oil on the skin before applying the poultice.

Another poultice that is popular in healing bursitis is one that is made from flaxseed or linseed. This is prepared by mixing a quarter pound of the crushed seeds with a pint of boiling water in a basin. After stirring until the mixture is like a smooth dough, add a half ounce of olive oil. When the mixture has cooled to a comfortable warmth, spread it onto linen, fold it over and apply to the painful area. A slightly different version uses a lesser amount of flaxseed, adding slippery elm powder and marshmallow in its place.

***Reflexology*** The technique of reflexology, with its focus on restoring the body's balance and promoting its healing, can be used as part of a treatment program for bursitis. Find the appropriate points on the hands or the feet that correspond to the location on the body where the bursitis is and try a combination of any reflexology techniques such as the finger walk, golf ball or thumb walk.

## Combining Treatments

The throbbing pain, acute tenderness and painful movement associated with bursitis are the key targets of any treatment plan, which can be arrived at in a number of ways. Over the years, many of the alternative and folk remedies used for healing bursitis have won acceptance not only among patients but also among allopathic and alternative practitioners alike. So, quite often there is a happy convergence of opinion regarding a particular alternative treatment or home remedy.

Since bursitis usually is not a serious condition, there is a fairly common belief among doctors that as long as the basic broad brush guidelines are being followed—i.e., rest and cold treatment in the beginning, heat and gentle exercise in the latter stage—any additional therapies that help reduce the pain and encourage healing are to be welcomed.

Most important for the acceptance of a technique, of course, is that the therapy does work to relieve the painful symptoms of bursitis and is not harmful or dangerous. The challenge is in trying to delineate which remedies to choose and how to fit them into any ongoing medical care.

## Table 5

| TREATMENTS FOR BURSITIS | |
|---|---|
| **Traditional** | **Alternative** |
| *RICE* <br> rest, ice, compression, elevation | *Acupuncture* |
| | *Castor oil treatment* |
| *Over-the-counter pain relievers* <br> aspirin; ibuprofen (Advil, Nuprin) | *Contrast treatments* <br> alternate hot, cold |
| *Nonsteroidal anti-inflammatory* <br> *drugs (NASAIDs)* | *Food therapy* <br> barley green; <br>    pineapple |
| *Corticosteroids* <br> local anesthetic used | *Homeopathy* <br> injection; oral; ruta <br>    grav; rhus toxico- <br>    dendron; benzoic <br>    acid; bryonia; <br>    Calcarea fluorica |
| *Fluid withdrawal* | |
| *Surgery* | |
| *Heat treatments* <br> heating pad; warm moist cloth | *Herbal tea* <br> chamomile; lady's <br>    slipper, skullcap; <br>    passion flower |
| *Ultrasound therapy* <br> *Exercise* | *Massage therapy* |
| | *Nutritional therapy* <br> calcium; magnesium; <br>    vitamins C, A, E |
| | *Poultices* |
| | *Reflexology* |

# CHAPTER 7

---

# Gout

Gout is a form of intense inflammatory arthritis, caused by the accumulation of deposits of small crystals of sodium urate in or around a joint, usually the big toe.

A disease that has been called the rheumatism of the rich and which to many people still is indelibly associated with the gluttonous indulgences of yesteryear's privileged nobility, gout has been a focus of treatment by doctors since Hippocrates. During the Middle Ages, European royalty often suffered from gout, which led many people to conclude that it was caused by a diet of rich foods and alcohol. History books describe famous and important dignitaries sitting at lavish banquets with their swollen feet resting on so-called gout stools, almost as a badge of honor. Famous patients have included Leonardo da Vinci, Martin Luther, Henry VIII, Charles Darwin, Alexander the Great and Benjamin Franklin. It is said that John Milton conveyed the intense suffering of his gout with the unrelenting horror in *Paradise Lost*.

The truth of the matter is that gout does not afflict only the upper classes. The normal level of uric acid does change regularly, based on your eating and drinking habits and a number of general health factors. At ordinary blood levels and even when slightly elevated, uric acid travels throughout the body in the bloodstream and is finally filtered out by the kidneys, then excreted in the urine. At higher levels of concentration, however, uric acid can accumulate and form sodium urate crystals, which are shaped like needles. These sharp crystals then deposit themselves in or around a joint, most frequently the big toe but sometimes in other small joints, especially the ankles, insteps, knees, elbows, wrists and fingers.

More than one million Americans have gout and 90 percent of them are men over forty. In women, gout usually occurs after menopause. About half of all gout patients are overweight, and 25 percent have a family history of the disorder. Gout does seem to strike with greatest frequency those men who are driven with ambition and considered successful on both economic and social levels.

In approximately two thirds of gout patients, the elevated levels of uric acid will occur because their bodies simply produce an excess amount of it. In the remaining third of patients, the elevated levels are a result of their bodies not eliminating uric acid in adequate amounts. It is believed that an inherited enzyme defect in the metabolic process that controls the production and elimination of uric acid is at fault. Curiously, though, most people who do have elevated blood levels of uric acid never develop the symptoms of gout. Ordinary occurrences such as dehydration and swallowing an aspirin can result in temporarily elevated uric acid levels.

Although the body does produce uric acid from substances call purines, which are found in many foods including kidneys, brains, meat extracts, dried beans, beer, sardines and anchovies, there is no evidence that most pa-

tients with gout regularly consume those foods that are rich
in purines. Normally, about one third of the uric acid in the
body comes from food and two thirds from normal metabolism. Alcoholic beverages will also increase uric acid levels.
A number of patients report that their attacks have followed
stress, fatigue, strenuous exercise, an infection, surgery, an
injury or overindulgence in alcohol or a particular food.

Gout may also appear as a complication of another, existing condition, such as leukemia, diabetes or lead poisoning.
Sometimes an attack is triggered by certain drugs—including penicillin, insulin, thiazide, diuretics and even modest
amounts of aspirin—that can interfere with the excretion of
uric acid.

Gout appears swiftly and painfully, without advance warning and often during the night. Typically, there is sudden and
severe pain in a small joint, most often the big toe because
the uric acid crystals tend to settle in parts of the body that
are located the furthest away from the center of the circulatory system, the heart. Within just a few hours, the joint is
swollen and extremely tender, and even the weight of a sheet
or blanket placed on it may be painful.

Sometimes there is an accompanying fever, and the inflamed skin over the joint will appear reddish and purple,
dry and shiny. This painful inflammation is caused by the
fierce battle that is underway between the sodium urate
crystals and the body's white blood cells, which come forward to attack the crystals. This battle triggers more crystals,
followed by additional numbers of white blood cells, creating in turn the throbbing inflammation.

The combination of sudden, intense pain and the accompanying inflammation very likely means a diagnosis of gout.
Sometimes an infection or trauma to a joint will seem like

gout to both patient and doctor alike. There are other conditions, however, that are similar in nature, including one called pseudogout. The symptoms of pseudogout are not as severe as actual gout and are actually caused by pyrophosphates rather than uric crystals. A diagnosis can be confirmed by laboratory testing for urate crystals in fluid removed from the affected joint.

An initial attack of gout that is left untreated most often will slowly subside over several days or weeks, and all outward signs will completely dissipate. For many people, that single attack will be a once-in-a-lifetime experience. However, we can expect that 50 percent of gout sufferers will have subsequent attacks, which tend to become more severe and occur more frequently. When urate crystals build up in joints over several years, they form lumpy deposits, a chalky white derivative of uric acid called tophi, which can severely damage joints. These attacks may affect a greater number of joints and, if left untreated, may result eventually in permanently deformed joints, high blood pressure and even life-threatening damage to the kidneys.

## Traditional Treatments

Although it isn't possible to prevent an initial attack of gout, much progress has been made over the years by the medical community in isolating the best strategies for coping. There are three areas of concern regarding gout: first, having the presence of the condition positively confirmed; second, treating the pain and inflammation of an attack; third, undertaking a strategy for minimizing the possibility of recurrent attacks.

An accurate diagnosis of the condition is crucial and easily accomplished by using a conclusive diagnostic test, first available in the 1960s, that isolates sodium urate crystals found in fluid removed from an inflamed joint. After the presence of gout as been confirmed, there are a number of medications that can treat an acute attack effectively, as well as other drugs that are available to prevent future occurrences.

## Responding to Acute Attacks

*Medication*   Although the standard medical treatment for acute attacks of gout consists of prescribing some form of anti-inflammatory drug, a number of unpleasant side effects have been associated with some of these medications.

Colchicine, a drug originally formulated from the autumn crocus, a common European plant, has been a powerfully effective treatment agent since the 1800s. Use of colchicine usually relieves pain and reduces the swelling of acute gout within forty-eight hours. However, colchicine often causes intestinal upsets, including nausea, vomiting, stomach cramps and diarrhea, when taken orally. Severe, even fatal blood disorders have resulted from intravenous use. Because it is so effective in counteracting an acute attack, many physicians will advise a patient to take colchicine hourly until the symptoms recede or until any of the side effects appear.

Indomethacin is a nonsteroidal anti-inflammatory drug (NSAID) developed in the 1950s that is highly effective in treating acute gout and is less toxic than colchicine. Naproxen is another NSAID that is also commonly used in treating acute gout.

If the NSAIDs fail to counter an attack, steroid drugs such as prednisone and adrenocorticotropic hormone may be prescribed, taken by mouth or by injection into the bloodstream or muscle.

For rapid relief of pain, your doctor might prescribe more powerful analgesics such as codeine or meperidine.

*Note:* The use of aspirin should be avoided because it can slow down the excretion of uric acid. Instead, your physician will probably prescribe ibuprofen or indomethacin.

**Bed rest**   It is important to keep weight off the affected joint, which most likely would feel less painful when propped up on a pillow or cushion. If the weight of sheets or blankets touching an afflicted joint causes pain, you can make a tent out of the bedding that will prevent it from touching the affected area.

**Preventative Medication**   It is possible to inhibit future attacks of gout through the use of preventive medication, which can be prescribed for use on an ongoing basis. These drugs work by lowering the level of uric acid in the blood so that crystals do not form. The treatment strategy will be based on an individual patient's metabolic history of either producing excessive quantities of uric acid or having an impaired ability to excrete it. Sometimes there's a combination of both conditions.

The excretion of uric acid can be increased by taking a uricosuric drug such as probenecid or sulfinpyrazone. Along with lowering blood uric acid levels, these drugs are also effective in dissolving any urate crystals that may have formed around the joints. There are possible side effects from these drugs, such as headache, nausea, upset stomach and a rash, so a trial and error of the right drug and level of dosage may be required to determine an appropriate treatment.

When there is an excessive production of uric acid, allopurinol is likely to be prescribed; it is an agent that slows down the rate at which uric acid is produced. Its side effects include a skin rash and upset stomach, as well as drowsiness in some people. Allopurinol may also have the more serious effect of altering the functioning of the liver, so patients should have routine blood tests on a regular basis.

## Alternative Treatments

*Acupuncture*   An acupuncturist treats gout by focusing on the dispersal of damp and heat, which are seen as having accumulated in the body. It is believed that the presence of damp is related to the failure of the spleen to process and distribute fluids effectively, while heat is believed to be related to dietary considerations. An acupuncturist would utilize points on the spleen channel to deal with dampness, while points on the liver and large intestine channels would be targeted to reduce heat and improve circulation of the *chi*.

*Aromatherapy*   It can be soothing to utilize fragrant, botanical oils during an acute occurrence. If the gout inflammation is lodged in your big toe, prepare a cool foot bath to which juniper and rosemary essential oils have been added, about ten drops of each oil to two quarts of cold water. In joints other than the foot, try making a soothing oil from one ounce of olive oil and five drops of juniper oil. Very gently massage the oil into the joint several times a day.

*Biofeedback*   Utilizing the technique of biofeedback can be useful as a long-range therapy for preventing future attacks. Utilize both deep breathing and biofeedback techniques to lower an elevated blood pressure. High blood pressure is not only unhealthy in and by itself, but many of the drugs that are prescribed to treat it will also elevate uric acid blood levels.

*Food therapy*   The focus of food therapy in treating gout is on avoiding foods that could trigger an attack. Certain foods that have a much greater concentration of purine are much more likely to induce gout and should be avoided. Included are kidneys, liver, heart, pork roast, sweetbreads, meat extracts, brains, gravies, anchovies and mussels.

Drinking lots of water is important because it can help to flush excess uric acid and also discourage the formation of kidney stones, which gout patients are prone to having. Drinking at least five or six glasses of water a day is recommended.

*Herbal tea*   A soothing cup of herbal tea is not only relaxing but is also an excellent way for a gout patient to increase consumption of fluids safely and pleasantly. While large amounts of fluid consumption are encouraged as a way of removing uric acid from the body, gout patients should avoid alcohol, because it is believed to increase uric acid production, while too much caffeine will render a patient jittery. A happy solution is herbal tea, which is soothing and contains no caffeine, alcohol or calories. Especially recommended are sarsaparilla, peppermint and yarrow.

*Herbal therapy*   The use of herbs, as prescribed by a herbalist, would necessarily be based on a personalized evaluation of the patient's entire health condition. Most frequently prescribed herbs for gout attacks include celery seed, which increases the removal of uric acid; willow bark, which acts as an anti-inflammatory; burdock, a generalized aid for improving the elimination of waste matter through the kidneys and bowels; silver birch, which increases the elimination of toxins and also reduces inflammation.

*Homeopathy*   Treatment by a homeopath is likely to focus on the ongoing factors in a patient's overall condition and lifestyle that perpetuate or trigger a gout condition as well as on ways to alleviate an acute attack. For example, were a patient to have an underlying state of health that was unsatisfactory, a homeopathic specialist might prescribe nux vomica as a way of strengthening the overall constitution and level of health, with the idea that the body would then be better able to combat the conditions that triggered gout. Along with nux vomica, a patient would also be given Ledum 30 to treat the specific symptoms of gout. Other symptom-specific homeopathic remedies include belladonna for red, hot and swollen joints; aconite for an acutely painful and red joint; colchicum for swelling in the big toe and Urtica urens for itching, burning and swelling.

*Hydrotherapy*   Water is very effective in giving instant relief from the throbbing pain of an acute attack. Ice and cold water treatments are recommended for up to twenty minutes at a time. Apply a cold, wet compress directly to the affected area or wrap an ice pack in a plastic bag and place it over a towel on the skin. Also soothing is a foot soak "flavored" with charcoal, which has the ability to draw toxins away from the body. An old bucket should be used because the charcoal will stain. In the bucket, just mix a half cup of charcoal powder with enough water to make a paste. Then, slowly add enough hot water to submerge your foot. A soak of a half hour to an hour should be plenty.

An alternate way of utilizing charcoal is by making a poultice. Use a blender to first grind a few tablespoons of flaxseed into meal. Mix that with a half cup of powdered charcoal and enough water, very warm, to make a paste. Apply the paste to the affected joint and use a cloth or plastic to hold it in place. Change it every four hours and be careful not to have the poultice touch clothing or bedclothes that are unprotected as it will stain.

***Reflexology***   Consult a reflexology chart to locate kidney point #25 on the soles of both feet, then use the techniques of rotation on a point and thumb walk. Rotation on a point is especially appropriate when the area is tender. With this method, use your index finger to apply pressure to the point and then rotate the hand being worked several times in a clockwise and then a counter-clockwise direction. In contrast, in the thumb walk, you use the outside edge of your thumb to burrow into the skin as the thumb takes tiny "steps," applying gentle and steady pressure all the while.

***Nutritional therapy***   Since obesity and an improper diet can increase the tendency for gout, nutrition is an important consideration in its treatment. A sensible diet that is low in fats and sugars can help to reduce extra pounds or maintain an appropriate weight. Meat should be avoided as much as possible because it contains large amounts of uric acid. Other foods that should be avoided include gravies; cakes, pies and any other foods that contain white flour and sugar products; dried beans; cauliflower; fish; lentils; oatmeal; peas; poultry; spinach and yeast products.

Also try to eliminate foods that are rich in purines, which cause an excess of uric acid. These foods include anchovies, asparagus, consommé, herring, meat gravies and broths, mushrooms, mussels, sardines and sweetbreads.

The cherry has developed a legendary power as a treatment for gout. A doctor confined to a wheelchair by severe gout accidentally discovered their healing benefits more than twenty years ago. After he wrote about his experiences and that of twelve other gout patients in a medical journal, the so-called "cherry solution" became a widespread treatment. Although there is no scientific explanation to account for it, others across the country have since found it works, consuming anywhere from ten cherries a day up to a half pound. It doesn't seem to matter whether the cherries are sweet or sour, or fresh, frozen or canned. One theory is that cherries are able to neutralize uric acid. Other dark red or blue berries have also been reported to be effective. Since those patients who have found success with cherries report virtually immediate results, you should try the cherries perhaps for a week and then discontinue if there is no improvement.

Vitamin supplements can play an active role for gout patients. It is generally believed that vitamin A and niacin can raise uric acid levels in the body, so intake of these two substances should be limited. Consumption of vitamin A on an ongoing basis should be no more than 5,000 IU daily and then none at all if you have an acute attack. Niacin, which you might be taking to help control cholesterol, should be limited to no more than 100 mg a day.

## Combined Treatments

Gout is an intensely painful condition that warrants immediate treatment when an acute attack occurs. While patients have a wide latitude in their individual tolerance for pain, the degree of discomfort associated with gout will test virtually anyone's tolerance. Most patients will want the immediate relief obtained from an anti-inflammatory drug. While there is no doubt that colchicine has been an effective agent of relief for more than one hundred fifty years, you would probably be wise to consider instead one of the NSAID drugs such as Indocin or another brand of indomethacin, which are less toxic. Along with the medication and bed rest, a topical treatment such as a cold pack or poultice would add soothing comfort at the very least.

After the initial attack has subsided, it is a far more challenging task to create an ongoing, lifetime strategy to deal with a gout condition. The typical gout patient is a male who is over forty, successful, overweight and often dealing with multiple frustrations in both his business and personal life. His lifestyle may include habits that could provoke another attack, such as an overindulgence in alcohol and protein, stress and working to a state of mental or physical fatigue. The initial attack of acute gout brings with it for many a life-altering wake-up call. These patients will look closely at their overall health and examine the elements in their lifestyle that are not conducive to wellness.

When a patient understands the basis of gout, that the body is either producing far too much uric acid or there's a problem in not getting rid of it fast enough, then the various treatments to be considered can be evaluated with one key objective in mind: how the treatment will help to lower the levels of uric acid in the blood so that urate crystals do not form.

Quite frequently, the gout patient is not in good overall health. Obesity, high blood pressure and a lack of physical fitness often go hand-in-hand with a gout condition. When told that gout can recur and be more severe, more frequent and more damaging, a patient who has just suffered through crippling pain will be in a more than usually receptive frame of mind to commit to an ongoing plan for preventing future attacks. Any ongoing plan will most likely center on the decision to commit to a daily medication to control the level of uric acid in the blood. Since the disease may be dormant for months or years after the initial attack, a physician may not want to prescribe ongoing drugs immediately. If the symptoms recur, however, sufferers will most likely need to discuss with their doctor the various factors involved.

If you choose to utilize ongoing medication, you'll first

need adequate testing to determine which of two drugs would be most useful. The uricosuric drugs, like probenecid and sulfinpyrazone, will increase the excretion of uric acid. However, if tests show that you are already excreting large amounts of uric acid, this drug would not be prescribed. The other drug, allopurinol, works to inhibit the formation of uric acid. In some instances, both drugs might be prescribed simultaneously. At the beginning of a long-term medication program, there is a possibility that the drugs themselves will induce an attack, so a very low dose of colchicine may also be prescribed during the first few months. You'll want to talk with your physician about any side effects that might be expected.

Along with a regimen of ongoing medication, a gout patient will benefit greatly from making lifestyle changes that will have a positive, overall effect on health. In addition to heeding traditional medical advice on restricting alcohol content, avoiding purine-heavy foods and eliminating excess weight, a gout patient should also consider complementary programs such as meditation, massage therapy and aromatherapy to reduce stress; homeopathy and acupuncture to strengthen the overall health and well-being.

There are gout patients who undergo substantial lifestyle changes and are able to attain improved states of health. You may not want to continue with an ongoing program of medication indefinitely, and you therefore may be a candidate for an alternative program of prevention or a modified version. Your physician will be able to help you decide, based on all that has been learned about your general condition, the underlying causes of your gout condition, the history of attacks and other factors about you.

## Table 6

### TREATMENTS FOR GOUT

#### Responding to Acute Attacks

| Traditional | Alternative |
|---|---|
| **Medication** <br> adrenocorticotropic (steroid drugs); codeine, colchicine; ibuprofen, meperidine, naproxen (NSAIDS); prednisone | **Acupuncture** <br> spleen, liver, large intestine channels targeted |
| **Bed rest** <br> propped pillows; elevated bedding | **Aromatherapy** <br> juniper/rosemary footbath |
|  | **Nutritional therapy** <br> limited fats and sugars; avoid meat, gravies, cakes, pies, white flour, sugar, dried beans, cauliflower, fish, lentils, oatmeal, peas, poultry, spinach and yeast |
|  | **Herbal tea** <br> sarsaparilla, peppermint, yarrow |
|  | **Herbal therapy** <br> celery seed, willow bark, silver birch |

*Table 6 (cont.)*

| Traditional | Alternative |
|---|---|
| | ***Homeopathy*** |
| | nux vomica, Ledum 30, belladonna, Colchicum, Urtica urens, aconite |
| | ***Hydrotherapy*** |
| | ice pack; cold compress; charcoal foot soak |
| | ***Reflexology*** |
| | kidney point #25 |

| **Taking Preventive Measures** | |
|---|---|
| Traditional | Alternative |
| ***Medication*** | ***Biofeedback*** |
| probenecid, sulfinpyrazone (uricosurics); allopurinol | blood pressure reduction |
| ***Lifestyle changes*** | ***Juice therapy*** |
| limited alcohol consumption; eliminate excess weight gradually; reduce stress | cherries added to diet |
| | ***Vitamin therapy*** |
| | vitamin A, niacin restrictions |

# CHAPTER 8

---

# Sprains and Dislocations

**A** weekend skier racing down the side of a mountain, a doctor stepping off a curb in high heel shoes and a Little Leaguer sliding into second base all are candidates for a painful joint injury such as a sprained ankle or dislocated shoulder.

There are more than one hundred joints in the human body, each one a well-designed structure of bone, ligament, tissue and cartilage that offers certain neighboring bones the ability to move in relation to one another. Joints can be categorized into three types, depending on the amount of motion allowed: rigid joints, like those in the skull or pelvis, are basically fixed and are movable only during infancy or pregnancy; slightly mobile joints, such as those between the vertebrae in the spine, which move only slightly but thereby create flexibility over the entire spinal column; and the freely mobile joints, as in the shoulders, knees, ankles, hips, fingers and toes.

Some freely mobile joints are hinged, which means that they move in just one plane, backward and forward, while others are ball-and-socket, moving backward and forward plus sideways. Typical hinge joints are fingers and elbows, while the shoulder and hip are examples of ball-and-socket joints.

If a joint is overflexed or forced to move in an unnatural direction, the ligaments, or the tissues that bind adjoining bones together, will be damaged. Since joints absorb the stress of movement, they are vulnerable to being wrenched and injured, especially in the case of the ankle and the knee. The degree of seriousness can range from injuries that are relatively easy to treat, such as a mild sprain, to much more serious traumas such as a joint dislocation that requires immediate medical treatment.

A sprain occurs when the ligaments are stretched too far or are actually torn, usually after a severe fall or a sudden and harsh twisting movement. The ligaments, which are fibrous bands of tissue that connect the bones, are designed to prevent excessive movement. In mild cases, the force of the injury affects only a few fibers of the ligament, resulting in mild to moderate pain and swelling that subside within a few days. A more violent injury may completely tear a ligament and require medical attention. Although any ligament can be sprained, it is the ligaments at the knees, ankles and fingers that are especially prone to injury, because greater force is more often applied to these joints.

The severity of a sprain can be classified as either mild, moderate or severe. A mild sprain is the result of fibers within the ligaments becoming overstretched or slightly torn. Minor pain is experienced and there is tenderness when the injured spot is touched or moved, but there is typically little or no swelling and some weight can be placed on the joint. In a moderate sprain, although the ligament fibers are torn they are not completely ruptured. Along with moderate pain and tenderness there will be some swelling and discoloration, and while movement of the joint is possible it is difficult and painful. A severe sprain has one or more ligaments that are completely torn and the affected area becomes painful, swollen, and black and blue. The joint cannot be moved normally or have any weight placed on it. When the sprain is so severe that all of the ligaments are torn, the joint may be misshapen as well as swollen.

A mild or moderate sprain can be self-treated with first-aid measures, but it may require medical attention if the pain continues for more than two or three days. Even medical professionals can have difficulty telling the difference between some sprains and fractures. A sprained wrist is nearly always x-rayed to see if it's been broken. If you're not certain as to the extent of the injury, it's best to treat a sprain as if it is a break until you can be certain. If you are able to hold a cup of tea in your hand after the injury, for instance, your wrist is probably not broken. A severe sprain should be examined at an emergency room as soon as possible to determine whether there is a fracture or a dislocation.

The dislocation of a joint is a serious and painful injury, usually the result of a violent trauma, such as a hard blow or sudden twisting force that occurs during a sports activity or a sudden fall. In a dislocated joint, not only have the ligaments been torn, but the bones that should be in contact with each other have been pulled apart so that there is a complete loss of contact and the joint no longer functions. There may also be damage to the joint capsule, the membrane that encases the joint, and there may be a fracture as well in one or both of the bones. In very severe cases, there may be nerve damage and some degree of paralysis as a result. A dislocated joint may look misshapen, is usually very painful and often is swollen, discolored and immovable.

About half of all dislocations happen to the shoulder, usually following a strong backward force striking an elevated arm. Other joints that are especially vulnerable to dislocations are those in the fingers, usually from being struck and bent backward; the elbow, after a hard fall on the arm or a forceful pull; the jaw, following a punch or other trauma to the mouth; the kneecap, where the knee can get twisted while scrambling down a steep incline.

In addition to being caused by a serious trauma, dislocation can also occur because of a complication of rheumatoid arthritis or because of a congenital defect. Also, when a joint has been weakened by an earlier injury, a dislocation may happen repeatedly in the future without an apparent cause. The jaw and shoulder joints are especially vulnerable to this kind of spontaneous dislocation.

If your joint is dislocated, it's very important to protect the injured area as best as you can and get to a doctor or a hospital as soon as possible. If it turns out that there is a fracture or other damage, it can be worsened if the injury is handled improperly.

## Traditional Treatments

*RICE*   Remember the acronym RICE, which summarizes the key elements of treatment for a sprain: rest, ice, compression and elevation. This treatment is very helpful in limiting the immediate pain, swelling and internal bleeding of the injury.

Resting the sprained ligament by immobilizing it will help to control the bleeding. Try to surround the injured joint with pillows or rolled-up blankets and keep it as still as possible for the first twenty-four hours. Limit your movement to the very minimum. For more severe sprains, an extended period of rest will probably be beneficial. A finger or toe can be immobilized by taping it to the digit next to it. A sling can be used to immobilize a sprained shoulder or elbow.

Ice applied to the injured joint as soon as possible is the most beneficial of the RICE components because it reduces swelling and inflammation. It's important to reduce swelling because swelling can damage cells by decreasing oxygen to the surrounding tissue. Application of cold slows down metabolism within the cell and allow tissues to survive the temporary lack of oxygen. This procedure speeds healing by promoting the renewal of cells. Cold also helps to relieve pain by numbing the area and preventing nerves from sending pain messages to the brain. Ice can be applied in a number of ways. However, it's important that the ice not be placed directly on the skin because that can cause frostbite or tissue damage. A bag of frozen vegetables from the freezer can function as an instant ice pack. Or, put some crushed ice in a plastic bag and wrap it in a towel or cloth. There are also instant, disposable cold packs that are chemically activated and last for about twenty minutes; reusable cold packs are first cooled in the freezer.

Apply the ice to the injury for no more than twenty minutes at a time because there's always the possibility of frostbite. Reapply every three or four hours during the first day or until there are no further signs of inflammation. It's all right for the area to be reddish and slightly numb, but if it turns white or blue, stop treatment immediately. And if you have a vascular disease, rheumatism or decreased sensation, speak to your doctor before applying ice.

Compression helps to decrease bruising and reduce the subsequent swelling of a sprained joint. Wrap the joint with strips of cloth in a figure-eight pattern, an Ace-brand bandage or other kind of elastic bandage. Don't wrap the injury too tightly, or the circulation may be cut off. The fit should be firmly snug but not tight. Use the figure-eight pattern for wrapping an ankle. For a wrist or ankle, be sure to leave the fingers or toes exposed and check periodically for signs of inadequate circulation, such as tingling, numbness, loss of motion or blue skin. If the bandage is too tight, remove it for fifteen minutes and then reapply it. Keep the injured area wrapped for three or four days.

Elevation of the injured area above the level of your heart will help to drain blood and fluids from the joint and thereby reduce swelling.

RICE, if undertaken promptly and continued for several days, will reduce the pain and swelling after the first twenty-four or forty-eight hours.

*Heat* Applications of heat can be undertaken once the pain and swelling have subsided, usually after the first forty-eight hours. Heat helps to prepare your muscles for strengthening exercises during rehabilitation. Apply heat for twenty minutes every three to four hours or as often as possible for the next few days. However, if the injury begins to swell again, immediately return to rest, ice, elevation and compression.

A hot compress can be prepared by soaking a cotton towel in hot water and then heating it in a microwave. If you cover the compress with a piece of plastic and a dry towel, the heat will be retained longer. A hot water bottle is very effective, filled halfway with hot or boiling water. If it feels too hot on the skin, then cover the bottle with a towel.

*Pain relievers* Aspirin or other over-the-counter remedies can be helpful in treating minor pain. If there is more severe pain, your doctor will probably prescribe stronger analgesics.

**Surgery**   In very severe cases, surgery may be needed to reconnect badly torn ligaments.

**Prompt professional medical care for dislocations**   Obtaining medical care quickly is essential and can prevent additional damage to blood vessels, tissues and nerves. It is important to get to a hospital or physician as quickly as possible. Be sure not to eat or drink anything because a general anesthetic may be required to have the dislocation repositioned during a surgical procedure. Afterwards, if the blood vessels, nerves and bones are in place and undamaged, the joint will probably be immobilized and put into a protective brace for two or three weeks until the other damaged tissues can heal.

## Complementary Treatments

Sprains

**Comfrey**   A poultice or compress applied to the joint can prevent inflammation, increase circulation and reduce pain. Comfrey became popular during the Middle Ages, when it earned the name of "knitbone" because of its ability to reduce swelling around fractures and promote bone unions. To make a comfrey poultice, mix three tablespoons of powdered root with three ounces of hot water, then stir into a paste. When cooled, apply the poultice to the skin and cover with sterile gauze, secured with a bandage. It can be left on for several hours or overnight. To make a comfrey compress, soak a cotton cloth or gauze bandage in an infusion, then cool the cloth and apply. Once a poultice or compress has been removed, massage the area with a salve or ointment containing comfrey.

*Herbal therapy*    Herbs provide a soothing aid for the healing of sprains. The herb arnica in any of its forms, including concentrate and tincture, is considered to be the most effective. Use five to ten drops of the concentrate applied directly to the area or a diluted form of the tincture, made by mixing one tablespoon of tincture per pint of cold water. Some people are allergic to arnica, so it's wise to test it on a small patch of skin. Also, don't apply to broken skin, because it could cause irritation.

Burdock, applied as a poultice or brewed as a tea, is an herb suggested for its soothing effect on sprained joints. Also recommended is a compress created by a tea brewed from the herb called dock. Ginger tea added to warm bath water creates a soothing soak.

*Acupressure*    The application of acupressure can help to relieve the pain of a sprained wrist or ankle. For a wrist, locate the hollow areas between the bones and tendons around the crease. Then, press firmly at the hollow area. On the ankle, find the large hollow that is in front of the large outer ankle bone and press that point.

*Food therapy*    Certain foods can aid in healing sprains, especially oranges, grapefruit, strawberries and peppers because of their high content of vitamin C. Vitamin C helps to mend collagen, the supportive protein in the skin, bones, tendons and cartilage, which can become damaged in a sprain.

*Ayurveda*    Practitioners of ayurveda emphasize the use of salt to relieve the swelling of a sprain. Combine one part salt and two parts turmeric mixed with enough water to make a paste. The paste should be applied to the sprained area once a day for twenty minutes to an hour. The paste should be covered with a cotton or muslin fabric to keep it from rubbing off and staining clothing. The skin itself may become discolored, but will wash off in several weeks.

**Homeopathy**  A homeopathic remedy can lessen the pain of a sprained joint. Within twenty-four hours of the injury, a dose of arnica 6 c is recommended. If that doesn't help or if the sprain feels better with slight movement rather than being immobilized, a dose of rhus toxicodendron 6 c is suggested. An alternative is ruta graveolens 6 c. These remedies can be taken as needed, but not more frequently than every two hours.

**Massage**  The swelling of a sprained joint can be reduced through massage. However, you need to wait at least forty-eight hours following the injury before using massage. A recommended technique is the rake massage. First place your hands on either side of the sprained joint. For the arm or wrist, you'll need to use just one hand, of course. Spread the fingers about a half inch apart and place the fingertips on the part of the joint that is farthest from the heart. For the knee, place the fingertips just below the knee, closest to the ankle. Then, pull the fingertips over the joint, applying light pressure, similar to using a rake. When you have gone past the top of the joint by a few inches, lift the hands and place them back at the starting point. This massage should be done for about five minutes at a time, several times a day.

**Herbal supplements**  There are a number of herbal supplements that can reduce inflammation and aid in healing. Bromelain, a natural enzyme derived from the pineapple, has been shown in several clinical studies to have anti-inflammatory and wound-healing properties. One theory says that bromelain breaks down fibrin, a blood protein that is part of the clotting process and allows for better tissue drainage and the reducing of localized pain and swelling. The recommended dosage of bromelain, which is available in 100-mg tablets, is 200 to 300 mg at the time of injury and 500 to 700 mg per day, taken between meals, for three to four days afterwards. Herbal practitioners suggest taking curcumin, the yellow pigment from the spice turmeric, along with bromelain as a way of increasing the anti-inflammatory effectiveness. The recommended dosage is 250 to 500 mg of curcumin with bromelain between meals.

*Nutritional therapy*   Nutritional supplements can help injuries heal. Recommended supplements and dosage include: three tablets of proteolytic enzymes daily; free-form amino acids, plus vitamin $B_{12}$ and vitamin $B_6$ and vitamin C; 1,500 to 2,000 mg of calcium daily; 750 to 1,000 mg. of magnesium daily; multimineral forma; 99 mg. of potassium daily; 500 silica daily; 100 mg. Vitamin B-complex daily; 5,000 mg. of Vitamin C daily; 500 IU of Vitamin E daily; and 50 mg. zinc daily.

*Reflexology*   The Technique of reflexology can be used in helping to heal sprained joints, working the reflex points on the hands or feet that correspond to the injured area. If you have a sprained knee, for example, try working the point 58 on the foot.

*Electrotherapy*   Using electrical muscle stimulation can help to maintain muscle mass and tone, by application of a very low dose of electrical current. This technique is especially beneficial when an injured joint is confined to a cast or is immobilized.

*Ultrasound*   An effective treatment of sprained joints makes use of ultrasound waves, which are vibrations that have the same physical nature as sound but with frequencies higher than the range of human hearing. These ultrasound waves heat the injured tissues and increase blood circulation.

*Yoga*  A recommended aid to healing sprained joints is yoga, because of its ability to boost circulation and trigger the body's relaxation mechanisms. Muscles are able to heal faster when they are in a relaxed state, which can be achieved through yoga as well as mental and emotional relaxation that is beneficial to the patient's sense of well-being.

*Menthol*  The application of menthol, when applied in a medicated gel, lotion or topical cream, can stimulate the nerve endings of muscles and create a cool sensation that temporarily eases the discomfort of a sprained joint. It also mildly numbs the nerve endings that register pain.

*Folk remedies*  There are a number of folk remedies that are successful in alleviating the discomfort of sprains. For instance, apply roasted onions or cut-up raw onions in the form of a poultice. Compresses made of apple-cider vinegar can be used to relieve pain. The inner surface of orange peel, taped or held against the injury, is said to reduce swelling. A mixture of one tablespoon of olive oil and five to ten drops of essential oil of wintergreen applied to the injury, then covered by a bandage, is supposed to relieve pain. A slice of cooled tofu is said to draw out heat more effectively than ice.

## Dislocations

*Homeopathy*  There are homeopathic remedies that can relieve pain and prevent the shock associated with the serious trauma of a dislocated joint. As soon as possible after the injury, take an oral dose of 6x or 12x arnica, repeated every half hour for three hours and then every three hours over the next three days. Arnica tincture or salve applied externally to the area will reduce swelling and bruising. Another recommended homeopathic treatment is rescue remedy, with a dose of three to four drops in a small glass of water sipped slowly and repeated every half hour until the patient is calm.

Several days after the injury, symphytum is suggested as an aid to help heal the injury. Recommended dosage of symphytum, which is prepared from comfrey, is 30c daily for three to four weeks.

**Herbal treatment**     Herbs can stimulate the healing of minor dislocations and damaged tissues. Comfrey is the most effective herb and is available in salves and ointments that can be rubbed directly into the skin. Also while more time-consuming and difficult to use than a salve, a comfrey poultice is probably stronger acting. A poultice can be made from three tablespoons of powdered comfrey root mixed with three ounces of hot water and stirred into a paste. This warm mixture can be applied directly to the skin, then covered with a sterile gauze cloth and secured with a bandage. The application can be left for several hours or overnight. After removing the poultice, massage the area with a comfrey ointment.

**Biomagnetism**     Healing with magnets is already popular in some European countries and in Japan, where a variety of products such as elasticized bandages with tiny magnets sewn in are available. In the U.S., an increasing number of scientists are now studying biomagnetism, defined as the use of extremely weak magnetic fields on the human body. Although biomagnetic devices presently are "nonapproved" for medical use in the United States, biomagnetic products are available to consumers through mail-order companies.

## Combined Treatments

Trauma injuries such as sprained joints and dislocated joints should receive immediate medical attention to prevent unnecessary additional damage. Except in the case of a very mild strain, it's always wise to have the joint treated by a physician. It is important to determine the full extent of the injury, which is not easily diagnosed without careful medical examination and, frequently, an X ray.

Immediately following the initial treatment by a physician, it's not only permissible but highly advisable to utilize the various healing alternatives that have been demonstrated to assist in the healing and to alleviate the pain and discomfort associated with such injuries.

### Table 7

## TREATMENTS FOR SPRAINS AND DISLOCATIONS

| Sprains | |
| --- | --- |
| **Traditional** | **Alternative** |
| *RICE* <br> Rest, ice, compression, elevation | *Comfrey* <br> poultice, compress |
| *Heat* | *Herbal therapy* <br> arnica; burdock; dock; ginger tea |
| *Pain relievers* <br> aspirin; analgesics | *Acupressure* |

*Table 7 (cont.)*

| Sprains | |
| --- | --- |
| **Traditional** | **Alternative** |
| *Surgery* | ***Food therapy***<br>oranges, grapefruit,<br>    strawberries, peppers |
| | ***Ayurveda***<br>salt, turmeric |
| | ***Homeopathy***<br>arnica; rhus toxicodendron;<br>    ruta graveolens |
| | ***Massage***<br>rake technique |
| | ***Herbal supplements***<br>bromelain; curcumin |
| | ***Nutritional therapy***<br>proteolytic enzymes; amino<br>    acids; vitamin $B_{12}$;<br>    vitamin $B_6$; Vitamin C;<br>    magnesium |
| | ***Reflexology*** |
| | ***Electrotherapy*** |
| | ***Ultrasound*** |
| | ***Yoga*** |
| | ***Menthol*** |

*Table 7 (cont.)*

| Sprains | |
| --- | --- |
| **Traditional** | **Alternative** |
| | ***Folk remedies*** <br> onions; vinegar; orange peel; tofu; oil of wintergreen |

| Dislocations | |
| --- | --- |
| **Traditional** | **Alternative** |
| ***Prompt medical care*** | ***Homeopathy*** <br> arnica; rescue remedy; symphytum |
| ***Physiotherapy*** | |
| | ***Herbal treatment*** <br> salves or ointments; comfrey poultice or compress |
| | ***Biomagnetism*** |

# CHAPTER 9

# Ankylosing Spondylitis: Inflammatory Back Pain

Ankylosing spondylitis is a form of inflammatory arthritis that affects the spine and sacroiliac joints. Spondylitis means inflammation involving joints of the spine and is derived from the Greek word for vertebra (*spondylos*) and inflammation (*itis*). As the inflammation subsides, healing takes place, with the bone growing out from both sides of the joint, eventually surrounding it completely. The joint is then unable to move and this stiffening is called ankylosis.

"Oh my aching back!" is the second most frequently heard medical complaint on earth, after the common cold, with 65 to 80 percent of the world's population suffering back pain at some time during their lives. Ninety percent of back pain is caused by the overuse of muscles or a trauma; it goes away on its own without any treatment. That's one reason why ankylosing spondylitis may go unrecognized for months or even years. The early back pain and morning stiffness of ankylosing spondylitis are often mistakenly treated as a form of back strain. Indeed, some people go through their lives with back complaints that are never correctly diagnosed as ankylosing spondylitis.

Nearly two million people in the U.S. have ankylosing spondylitis, a disease that's been around at least three thousand years, with evidence of its presence having been observed in some Egyptian mummies. It generally strikes people in their late adolescence or early twenties, and men tend to be afflicted about twice as often as women. This form of inflammatory arthritis is included in a family of diseases called spondylarthropathies, which attack the spine. In addition to ankylosing spondylitis, these diseases include Reiter's syndrome, some cases of psoriatic arthritis and arthritic inflammatory bowel diseases.

The cause of ankylosing spondylitis is still unknown, but all of the spondylarthropathies do share a common genetic marker, the white cell blood group that is numbered HLA-B27. Ankylosing spondylitis is three hundred times more common in people who have the HLA-B27 gene than among those who do not. This means that virtually all people with ankylosing spondylitis will have HLA-B27. However, the reverse is not true. All people with the HLA-B27 marker will not have ankylosing spondylitis. Indeed, there are far more people with the blood group who will never get ankylosing spondylitis than there are people who do get it: it is estimated that more than 95 percent of those who are HLA-B27 positive never develop the disease. The HLA-B27 gene occurs in 7 to 10 percent of populations of European origin and appears much less frequently in African and Japanese populations. However, the gene can occur as high at 50 percent in North American Indian populations.

Since the gene runs in families, it is not unusual for more than one family member to have the disease. In fact, over one half of patients with ankylosing spondylitis have another family member who has the disease. The HLA-B27 gene does not cause ankylosing spondylitis, but people with the gene are more susceptible to getting the disease. It is believed that an intestinal infection from one or more unknown bacteria may trigger ankylosing spondylitis in susceptible people. Researchers are at work trying to identify which bacteria are involved. In some cases, the disease has occurred in those predisposed people after exposure to bowel or urinary tract infections.

Symptoms of ankylosing spondylitis usually begin in late adolescence or early adulthood, at approximately twenty to twenty-five years of age. Often, the symptoms are ignored, attributed to growing pains or youthful exertion. Typically, ankylosing spondylitis originates in the sacroiliac joints, where the vertebrae of the spine meet the pelvis. The most common and early complaint is chronic lower back pain that starts gradually and persists for more than three months rather than coming in attacks. This back pain is dull in character and is felt primarily deep in the gluteal region and lower part of the back during the early stages. There is also stiffness in the back that is worse in the morning and then eases after mild physical activity or a hot shower. There may also be pain and stiffness after a prolonged period of sitting, for example, in a movie theater or on a long car ride.

These symptoms are in contrast to the symptoms of back pain that occur as the result of mechanical causes, which include: a sudden rather than gradual onset; pain that is localized across the lower back; usually no stiffness in the morning; the onset of symptoms occurring at any age, with a kind of back pain that usually is made worse by exercise but that can be relieved by prolonged bed rest.

Ankylosing spondylitis produces an ache that is felt in the buttocks and, sometimes, down the backs of the thighs and in the lower part of the back. One side is commonly more painful than the other and arises from the sacroiliac joints. The disease tends to progress from the lower back up to the vertebrae in the neck. Pain is not always confined to the back. Some patients have chest pain, which worsens on deep breathing and is felt around the ribs. This chest pain does not come from the heart but from the joints between the ribs and the backbone. For many, it feels difficult to move the ribs fully when breathing deeply, although the lungs can continue to work because the diaphragm is not affected. In severely affected patients, when the rib cage does not move well, pneumonia can develop.

Sometimes, either at the beginning or later on, ankylosing spondylitis may affect joints other than in the spine, including the shoulders, hips, knees, ankles and feet. Also, certain tender places may develop in bones that are not part of the spine. One of these is the heel bone, which makes it uncomfortable to stand on a hard floor, and another is the bone of the seat, making hard chairs unpleasant. In approximately one out of seven patients, attacks of inflammation of the eye will occur.

There is no diagnostic test that can be given at the onset of back pain to confirm the presence of ankylosing spondylitis. A description of the patient's symptoms, which differ from those of mechanical back pain, should alert the doctor to consider that a patient may be developing ankylosing spondylitis. Additionally, identification of the HLA-B27 gene factor would provide additional positive data for consideration. In addition to taking a history of symptoms, the doctor will examine the patient, looking for muscle spasm and noting posture and mobility in the back, along with reviewing other parts of the body for evidence of the disease.

A diagnosis of ankylosing spondylitis can be confirmed from an X ray taken of the sacroiliac joints, if these reveal changes in tissues that are caused by inflammation. However, these tissue changes don't always appear on X rays during the early stages of the disease. The doctor will also probably test for anemia and perform a test called the erythrocyte sedimentation rate (ESR), which tells how active the disease is.

Since early treatment is critical to reduce uncontrolled inflammation and pain and to prevent long-term deformities, an experienced physician will often diagnose the disease and begin treatment even before the x-ray findings are conclusive, relying on symptoms, the presence of the HLA-B27 gene and the physical examination.

No two cases of ankylosing spondylitis are exactly the same, the disease takes a different course in different people, and the symptoms may come and go over long periods. But eventually ankylosing spondylitis becomes less severe. However, the lumbar spine usually becomes stiff and the upper part of the back and the neck can stiffen as well. The worst disability resulting from ankylosing spondylitis is fixation of the back in a bent or stooped position. This used to be quite common in ankylosing spondylitis patients but is now prevented by early diagnosis and treatment.

Over time, the inflammation at the ends of the ligaments results in stiffness, and movement becomes painful. After a period of stiffness and pain, a bony bridge grows between the parts, and the area becomes totally rigid. This fusion stops motion but has the beneficial effect of eliminating pain since pain is experienced only in areas that are still able to move.

In contrast to rheumatoid arthritis, which can cause destruction of the bones around a joint, ankylosing spondylitis fuses the intact bones together. This bony fusion can be extensive in the most severely affected patients and can lead to the creation of a single giant bone that includes the pelvis, the spine, the skull and the ribs, leaving the central part of the body without any motion at all. People who do develop a stiff or "ankylosed" spine will nevertheless remain functional if this fusion occurs in an upright position. Probably the most common significant limitation is a fusion of the neck in a flexed position, which limits the person's ability to raise the head.

## Traditional Treatments

Since there is no cure for ankylosing spondylitis, the doctor will aim to relieve the symptoms, improve spinal mobility where it may have been lost and help a patient pursue a normal occupational and social life. Although the disease tends to become less active in later years, the treatment really continues forever. In addition to taking medication for the relief of pain and inflammation, a patient will need to incorporate physical therapy, exercise, diet, rest and posture control into a daily routine. This combination of anti-inflammatory medication and a sustained program of exercise can slow down the progression of the disease and enable the patient to maintain activity.

*Drug treatment*   As a way of relieving any pain and inflammation, helping to get a good night's sleep and gaining sufficient freedom from pain to take part in an exercise program (another critical element of successful therapy), drug treatment can be an important element in any treatment plan for patients with ankylosing spondylitis. Nonsteroidal anti-inflammatory medications (NSAIDs) generally provide the most effective results. Indomethacin is most commonly prescribed, and is available in a suppository to counter early morning stiffness. Because it has serious side effects, phenylbutazone is used only when other NSAIDs have failed.

Many patients find that they need continuous treatment on a small maintenance dose of their drug. Some of the newer tablets are manufactured to remain effective throughout the night and into the first part of the day.

*Good posture*      An important element of an ongoing treatment program for ankylosing spondylitis is the maintenance of good posture, in order to prevent progressive stooping from flexion of the spine. Although it is rare for the spine to stiffen completely, a conscious effort towards maintaining good posture will ensure that if it does happen, at least it stiffens in an erect rather than a bent position. You must develop the habit of being aware of your posture and being sure to correct it constantly, not only during exercise periods but throughout the day, while standing, sitting and walking.

At home, to maintain good posture while sitting, select a chair that has a firm seat, straight back and armrests. There should be firm rather than soft padding on the seat and back. The seat of the chair should not be too long from front to back because this will make it difficult to place your lower spine into the base of the back of the chair. Don't sit for long in low, soft chairs, as this will result in bad posture and increased pain.

At the office, pay special attention to the position of your back so that you do not have to stoop. Make sure that your seat is at the proper height and do not sit in one position for too long without moving your back. A job that allows a variety of movements—sitting, standing and walking—is ideal. Most unsuitable would be a job where you would have to stoop or crouch over a table or a computer console for hours at a time. If you do have a job that keeps you in one place for long periods of time, make sure you get up at least every hour and stretch and walk around. It would be ideal to be able to lie flat for fifteen minutes at midday.

If you have to make a long journey in a car, it's very important to stop for five minutes every hour or so and get out of the car for a stretch. This is not only beneficial for maintenance of your posture, it's also a safety factor since pain and stiffness can distract your attention from driving. Patients who have stiffness of the neck and other parts of their spine have difficulty backing into parking spaces because they can't turn easily to look behind them. Special mirrors are available to fit onto your car that can help. Headrests for the front seats are also advised so that sudden deceleration injuries to the neck can be avoided. A stiff neck is more easily hurt than a normal neck.

When lying in bed, it is important to be flat on your back; also practice lying face down some of the time. This prone lying, as it is called, should be done for twenty minutes in the morning and twenty minutes before going to bed at night. At first, you might not be able to tolerate more than five minutes of prone lying at a time or perhaps you may need a pillow under your chest. With practice, as the spine relaxes, it becomes easier. Making a habit of this will help to prevent your back and hips from becoming bent.

The bed you sleep on should be firm, without a soft or sagging mattress. A sheet of plywood or chipboard two feet by five feet by one half inch is ideal to place between the mattress and the bed frame. Not only is a firm bed more comfortable to lie on than one that is yielding, but it will help prevent any tendency for spinal curvature to develop later on.

***Physical therapy***   In order to maintain mobility of the joints affected by ankylosing spondylitis, regular physical therapy is vital. Ideally, a physical therapist, in consultation with your doctor, will design an exercise routine tailored to your individual requirements. Once you have learned the exercises, try to do at least some of the routine, if not all of it, every day. Exercise helps to make you conscious of your posture, especially the position of your back, and also encourages free movement of certain joints, especially the shoulders and hips. It is important to keep muscles strong, because reduced movement, even for a short time, allows them to become weaker, and it takes a long time to build them up again. Here are some suggested exercises:

1. Standing with your heels and seat against a wall and keeping your chin in, push your head back towards the wall and keep it back for the count of five, then relax. Repeat ten times.
2. Sit on a firm chair, put your right hand across your chest and hold the side of the chair. Stretch your left arm out in front of you and then twist to the left, taking the arm horizontally as far behind you as possible, turning your head to look over the left shoulder. Hold this position, then push and turn a little further, hold that position and then return to facing forward. Repeat three times with each arm.

3. Sit with your shoulders relaxed and chin drawn in, looking straight ahead. Bend your head sideways to bring your right ear toward your right shoulder, hold it here, make sure your shoulder muscles are still relaxed and bend a bit further, then return to straight. As you do the side bending, the profile of your nose should remain in the same place, to make sure you don't turn your head. Repeat, bending to each side twice.

   Now tip your head back, looking up the wall and along the ceiling and bring it back to straight. Repeat.

   Change to tipping your head forward as far as possible to get your chin touching your neck, and return to straight with chin pulled in. Repeat once.

4. Lie on your back with knees bent up, lift up your hips so your seat is off the floor and there is a straight line from shoulder to knees. Hold for the count of five, and lower. Repeat five times.

5. Lie on your stomach, head turned to one side, hands by your sides. If necessary, you may put a pillow under your chest, but not at your waist, in order to get comfortable. Raise one leg off the ground, keeping your knee straight. Repeat five times with each leg, making sure your thigh comes off the ground.

   Raise your head and shoulders off the ground as high as you can ten times.

6. Kneeling on the floor on all fours, lift and stretch the opposite arm and leg out parallel with the floor and hold for the count of ten. Lower and then repeat with other arm and leg. Repeat five times each side.

7. Lie on your back with your legs straight. Put your hands on your ribs at the sides of chest. Breathe in deeply through your nose and out through your mouth, pushing your ribs out against your hands as you breathe in. Repeat ten times. Remember, it is as important to breathe out fully as it is to breathe in deeply.

   Put your hands on the upper part of the front of your chest. Breathe in deeply through your nose and then breathe out as far as you can through your mouth. Push your ribs up against your hands as you breathe in. Repeat ten times.

Sports should be an important element of your physical therapy program. The ideal sport for an ankylosing spondylitis patient is swimming, since it uses all the muscles and joints without jarring them. Contact sports are not ideal, because the joints can get injured. Golf has drawbacks, because players may spend long periods putting, during which the spine is in continued flexion. Basketball and volleyball are excellent, as they combine movement with stretching and jumping. Another excellent activity is cycling, because it helps to keep the joints active and strengthens the muscles in the legs. It also provides good breathing exercise and helps the rib cage continue to expand. Be sure that the handlebars of the bicycle are adjusted so the rider is sitting tall, not hunched over.

***Surgical procedures*** Surgery is occasionally used in correcting late spinal deformities in the back or neck when they are so severe that the patient cannot look forward and has difficulty crossing the road. This operative treatment may not be possible in some instances, though, because of the difficulty of safely giving anesthesia in a patient with severe ankylosing spondylitis. Total hip replacement is a more frequent surgical treatment, for a patient who has become disabled by deterioration of the joint.

***Adaptive aids and devices***    Patients who face severe lifestyle restrictions in the wake of irreversible deformities can facilitate the performance of many activities through the use of specially designed adaptive aids and devices. For example, when the neck and back are flexed so far forward that walking and reading are difficult, prism glasses can improve the field of vision. Ambulation aids, such as canes, can also help to maintain activity and prevent falls. Special rearview mirrors can be installed on automobiles to help increase visibility for patients who drive. A contoured cervical pillow and lumbar-roll cushion can help patients maintain good posture while sleeping.

***Counseling***    In a long-range treatment program for a person with ankylosing spondylitis, counselors, including specialists in physical therapy and occupational therapy, can help fashion the kinds of exercise programs and adaptive adjustments that will make life more manageable. Also, by joining ankylosing spondylitis patients' groups, sufferers can gain emotional support, accurate information and greater understanding of the disease.

***Diet***    A treatment program for ankylosing spondylitis should include an emphasis on good nutrition and weight control. The latter is important for maintaining overall good health and energy as well as for protecting the joints from the strain of added weight. Recommended daily are two helpings of protein food, fruits, vegetables and other foods that are the source of vitamins and calcium.

*Heat* The pain and stiffness of ankylosing spondylitis in the spine and neck can be alleviated by the application of heat. A hot bath before retiring or a hot water bottle or electric blanket in bed are usually adequate.

## Alternative Treatments

The traditional approach to treating ankylosing spondylitis is an ongoing, multifaceted treatment program, combining medication, physical therapy, exercise, diet and posture control. Since a patient must plan on continuing treatment over a lifelong term, the incorporation of alternative methods within the program can help to add variety and interest.

Certain mainstays of alternative healing, however, should be avoided. For example, spinal manipulation should not be undertaken, as there is a real danger of severe harm occurring to the spinal column.

Most beneficial to ankylosing spondylitis patients are those therapies that emphasize relaxation of tensions, relief from pain and maintenance of a positive outlook.

*Alexander Technique* A philosophy emphasizing the need to relearn the natural body posture that one was born with and that has been undone over the years through stress, improper breathing and general abuse of posture is the Alexander Technique. No manipulation of the spine is involved, with the emphasis being on posture and breathing, so the technique should be safe for ankylosing spondylitis patients. Before consulting with an Alexander teacher, however, you should talk with your doctor and see if there are any restrictions you should know about.

*Relaxation techniques* There are daily tensions that tighten up muscles and even the ability to breathe deeply, which can exacerbate efforts to maintain good posture. Relaxation techniques can loosen muscles and smooth breathing. Try techniques such as meditation, music, etc., until you find one that works best for you.

## Combined Treatments

When faced with maintaining a treatment program for a chronic, incurable disease like ankylosing spondylitis over a period of perhaps thirty or forty years, it's very important to keep your daily routine fresh and appealing, especially the elements of your daily exercise program, because the persistence of your efforts is directly related to long-term success in lessening deformities. Therefore, you must see your doctor regularly to maintain an accurate gauge of how well things are working and what changes ought to be made.

Also, it's very important to keep up-to-date with the latest findings in research, treatment options and the experiences of other patients. Just applying on a daily basis all of the traditional therapies that are advised for an ankylosing spondylitis patient will leave little time in the day to add alternative treatments. However, when a highly praised technique does seem worth trying, discuss it with your doctor to see how you might best try it out.

## Table 8

# TREATMENTS FOR ANKYLOSING SPONDYLITIS

| Traditional | Alternative |
|---|---|
| **Drug treatment** | **Alexander Technique** |
| NSAIDs: indomethacin; phenylbutazone | **Relaxation techniques** |
| **Good posture** | |
| lying prone, firm chairs, regular stretching | |
| **Physical therapy** | |
| exercise program; swimming; sports; bike riding | |
| **Surgical procedures** | |
| correction of deformities; total hip replacement | |
| **Adaptive aids and devices** | |
| prism glasses; canes; rear view mirrors; cervical pillow; lumbar cushion | |
| **Counseling** | |
| therapists; support groups | |
| **Diet** | |
| good nutrition; weight control; daily protein foods, fruits, vegetables, vitamins, calcium | |
| **Heat** | |
| hot bath; electric blanket; hot water bottle | |

# CHAPTER 10

---

# Bunions

The bunion, a highly visible malady of the foot that is virtually impossible to ignore, is misunderstood by many people. For example, it's a widely held belief that bunions are caused by wearing high heels. Actually, a bunion is caused by an abnormal walking pattern, which in turn is the result of incorrect biomechanics, the function or mechanics of a living body. In the case of a typical bunion patient, the excessive pronation causes a deviation to form in the joint of the big toe, creating a *hallux valgus*, or more commonly known as a bunion.

This conspicuous bump on the affected big toe looks unsightly and becomes painful when irritated by shoes that cannot conform to the shape of the protrusion. While not the cause of the bunion, shoes definitely can exacerbate the problem and cause discomfort when they are tight fitting.

The biomechanics of the human gait focuses on how the body weight is distributed as the feet come in contact with the ground and then on through the weight-bearing phase of the stride.

With twenty-six bones, thirty-three joints and more than one hundred tendons, muscles and ligaments, the human foot is an engineering marvel that most of us take for granted—until something goes wrong. And it does go wrong: at least 75 percent of Americans experience a foot problem of some degree of seriousness during their lives. Even so, it's typical to ignore early warning signs, because people seem to think that aches and pains in their feet are something to be expected.

Bunions and other big-toe problems are caused by excessive pronation during the early, toe-off phase of the gait, when the foot is about to leave the ground and is pushing off. Pronation is an inward rolling of the foot, which puts pressure on the area where bunions tend to develop. People with flat feet or low arches are most likely to pronate and therefore most likely to end up with bunions.

Many people have biomechanical abnormalities but never suffer any discomfort at all. For some reason, the imperfections in their walking gait do not translate into problems like bunions.

High heels are especially brutal on bunions because they force the toes drastically towards the inside when the forefoot is in the weight-bearing phase of the stride. This then creates enormous stress on the big-toe joint. For example, a woman who is walking in three-inch heels will have her weight shift almost directly from her heel to the ball of her foot. During that shift, her midfoot bears virtually no weight at all during the stride. This is not normal and places tremendous extra pressure on the ball of her foot, and therefore on the metatarsal bones. It is the combination of the excessive pressure on the big-toe joint and on the head of the first metatarsal bone, along with the shoe's too-small toe box, that squeezes the cramped toes; added to the abnormal biomechanics, all contribute to the development of bunions.

In addition to a tendency to overpronate, the typical bunion patient may very well have a genetic tendency to develop the disorder because of an inherited foot structure. In fact, bunions can be genetically traced in 30 percent of the patients who have them. Certain foot shapes have been found to be more likely than others to develop bunions. So, for instance, a person with a long big toe might be a prime candidate for a bunion because greater leverage is exerted on it during walking.

Although both men and women of all ages can develop bunions, a woman is much more likely to develop this condition. A survey by the American Podiatry Association of 218 female patients aged forty and over confirmed that bunions are indeed a common affliction since all of the women reported having the condition in either a mild or severe form, ranging from a mild inflammation to permanent bone deformity. This high incidence of bunions occurring in women is due to the long-term wearing of traditional, fashionable shoes that feature high heels and a narrow toe box. Men, by contrast, have shoe styles that rarely change, with heel heights in the one-inch range and a wide range of shoe sizes and widths that emphasize comfort.

Thus, the combination of a genetic disposition, faulty biomechanics and unfriendly shoes over a period of time can result in a sizable bunion condition. Actually, there are two types of bunions, which are defined by the stage of the condition. The acute bunion, which is accompanied by a noticeable and sometimes sharp pain, develops from a bursitis. Bursitis is an inflammation of a bursa, a sac containing tissue fluid, located at the big toe joint and serving as the lubricant between the skin and the bones.

Continued irritation of the skin by an ill-fitting shoe causes the sac to become inflamed and inflated with more fluid, resulting in acute bursitis. This acute condition can then develop, over time, into the painless but full-fledged deformity known in medical nomenclature as hallux valgus. This happens as the bursal fluid begins to solidify into a mass that resembles gelatin, a process further stimulated by pressure upon the joint resulting from the foot being pressed into shoes that cannot accommodate the ball of the foot; with its burgeoning bunion growth, the ball is now disproportionally wider than the heel. This condition worsens when high-heeled shoes are worn because in order for the shoe to stay on the foot, it must fit snugly at the heel. Since the ball of the foot is wider, the shoe with a snug heel that prevents slippage generally will not accommodate the expanding width of the ball of the foot at the front of the shoe. This improper fit at the ball of the foot leads to the increasing angulation of the big toe joint and the deformity of hallux valgus.

Hallux valgus is a serious condition because it strains the foot and produces an abnormal prominence of the joints. As a result of the widening of the front of the foot through the bunion condition, there is a loss of balance. The growing deformity of the big toe will begin to affect simple movements of standing and walking. There is the possibility of arthritis developing as a result of the condition.

As hallux valgus progresses, the tendons of the toes begin to shorten, the muscles contract and eventually nearly all of the bones located in the front of the foot are displaced. The big toe will continue to angulate more and more until it lies across or under the second toe, which can lead to another problem known as "hammertoe." However, there is no pain at this stage, so it is quite common for little or no attention to be given to the problem. Most people will not do anything about a bunion until the condition becomes painful again. Typically, this happens when the patient is over fifty, after years of continued aggravation of the condition, although it can occur earlier. The pain most likely will come not from the bursitis but from osteoarthritis or from corns and calluses that form at the site of the friction and the pressure. At this point, the deformity of the joint might be permanent, in which case two options are available. One is to have the protruding part of the bone removed by surgery and the other is to accommodate the deformed joint by larger shoes and special devices such as rubber toe shields.

## Traditional Treatments

There are two distinct courses of treatment for bunions: preventive and corrective. Preventive methods are aimed at preventing or delaying the continued worsening of a bunion, while corrective techniques, usually of a surgical nature, aim at curing the disorder.

Preventive measures are useful from the time that a person's abnormal pronation has been identified, well before any symptoms appear or at the time when the earliest beginnings of a bunion have taken form. Many of the preventive measures are pragmatic, very simple to employ and often successful in preventing advanced deformity of the joint.

*Footwear*  The most important factor in the development of bunions is the style and fit of the shoe, which ultimately aids or prevents a progression from the acute bursitis stage to a full-blown chronic bunion deformity. The effect of footwear on bunions has been dramatically demonstrated over the years.

When shopping for a shoe, consider the following tips. First, remember that any shoe with a pointed toe box will cram your toes together. Look for shoes that combine a wider, not pointed, toe box and a narrow heel base. Use the following test to determine the proper fit. Remove the right shoe, then place the sole of the left foot on the bottom of the right shoe. If the foot hangs over the side of the shoe, it's not the right fit. Also, trace the outline of one foot on a large piece of paper, and then cut around the tracing. Put your shoe on the paper cut-out. If the shoe is larger than the tracing, particularly in the front, the shoe does not fit.

Enormous progress has taken place in the design and production of athletic shoes, resulting in shoes so comfortable that 90 percent of the running shoes sold today are bought by nonrunners. What's particularly beneficial about today's athletic shoes is that they are soft and lightweight and they contain excellent shock absorption. The shoes are also designed to keep the foot in the flat position, which helps to prevent abnormal pronation.

There is also a design emphasis on achieving solid stability, which helps prevent overpronation. Many athletic shoes have a stabilizing bar in them, located on the inside part of the heel where overpronation often occurs. Cross trainers are probably the best shoes for a bunion because of the shock absorption contained in the forefoot, along with the built-in flexibility for a wide range of foot motions.

**Heating pad**   The use of a heating pad applied to a bunion on a regular basis will increase the blood flow, which can help to break up the inflammation.

**Orthotics**   There are inserts for shoes that are designed to improve your walk. Called orthotics, mass-produced ones are sold mainly by athletic stores; there are also custom-fit, prescription models. Custom orthotics are created from a cast impression of your feet, and they incorporate the corrections a podiatrist has found necessary after analyzing the way you walk. Most are made from thermal plastics. Unlike corrective shoes, which stop pain but limit movement, orthotics enhance movement by positioning the foot so it can support itself.

Orthotics are especially good for bunions because they

properly balance the distribution of weight on the foot when it comes in contact with the ground. If a biomechanical problem is diagnosed early enough, the use of orthotics can prevent the need for any future corrective surgery. And in the case of those who do undergo the latest form of bunion surgery (see below), the use of orthotics afterwards will almost completely assure the prevention of any recurrence of the bunion.

A new pair of orthotics requires a special wearing schedule. They must be broken in safely, because it takes a while for your body to become accustomed to walking differently; overuse at the beginning is likely to bring on aches and pain throughout the lower extremities. Orthotics should be worn for only an hour or two the first day, followed by a gradual increase in each of the following days until they can be left in the shoes all day.

**Pads**   A moleskin pad can cushion a bunion and the accompanying calluses on the bottom of the foot. Moleskin is a feltlike material made from sheep's wool; the pads come in self-adhesive sheets that can be cut to fit over sensitive areas on the foot that are prone to friction, including the joint of the big toe.

**Separation**   The big toe can be separated from the second toe with a quarter-inch-thick foam rubber pad, put in place at bedtime, which can help to keep toes in alignment and prevent recurrence of a bunion.

**Sling pad**   An over-the-counter product called a sling pad can be used to pull the big toe away from the second toe and take pressure off the bump.

**Surgery**   Surgery may become necessary if the condition reaches the point where a patient is experiencing continual pain and the bunion is interfering with walking and other activities. Surgical techniques for correcting bunions were first described in medical literature more than one hundred years ago. These techniques ranged from amputation of the big toe to variations of treatments that were used on hands. Virtually all of the techniques, except for amputation, failed to correct the underlying problem, and the bunion would usually reappear after a few years.

Over the years, many improvements have been made in surgical techniques for bunions, along with the cessation of amputation as a recommended method. However, up until a few years ago, the techniques still did not correct the cause of the condition. Now there are surgical procedures that incorporate the realignment of the bone with the correction of the abnormal motion that led to the deformity.

When a chronic bunion deformity has begun to interfere with daily life, surgery may be necessary. Until recently, surgery was performed to realign the bones so that the bump was removed and the toe looked normal. However, after the operation, the pressure would continue because the excess pronation had not been corrected. As a result, the first metatarsal bone would eventually be pulled out of alignment and a new bunion would form. Now, surgical procedures have been devised that not only move the bones into proper alignment but also slide the first metatarsal bone downwards into a normal position, which can then help to prevent the overpronation that causes formation of a bunion.

There are two surgical approaches that are commonly used, the open and the closed techniques.

Open bunion surgery utilizes a large open wound, with a three-to-six-inch incision, through which the sesamoid bones, small modular bones that develop in a joint or tendon, are removed, the tendons are lengthened, a wedge of bone is removed from the metatarsal, and any arthritic spurs that produce bony bulges are excised. Additionally, the joint capsule is cut and the remaining structures are wired into place. This kind of operation is usually performed in a hospital; it may require a week's stay and is then followed by several months of rest with the patient wearing a nonwalking cast.

Closed bunion surgery utilizes an incision that is smaller than one-half inch and often takes place on an outpatient basis. After part of the bony protuberance is removed, the large toe is repositioned and held in place with an adhesive dressing that is worn for about three weeks; complete healing takes six to eight weeks. The patient is able to leave the ambulatory foot surgeon's office wearing a surgical shoe rather than a cast.

Both types of procedure are serious, because soft tissue is being traumatized and bone is being cut or shaved. They produce significant swelling and discomfort, along with the danger of infections occurring during the healing process. Making the decision to have surgery is not easy nor is it easy deciding whether to entrust your feet to an orthopedic surgeon or a podiatrist. There are both podiatrists and orthopedic surgeons who are trained to perform bunion surgery. Some specialize in the open method, while others in both groups specialize in the closed method, with those who are skilled in both procedures. Talk to people who have had the procedures performed and find out what their experience has been, both immediately afterwards and long-term.

## Alternative Treatments

If you have a bunion, most likely you will want to look for techniques that will minimize the pain and relieve any inflammation. At the earliest stages of a bunion, the primary goal is to prevent it from progressing to a chronic deformity that will involve a permanent rigidity of the bones. And if you've had bunion surgery already, it's important to put into practice those therapies that will prevent any reemergence of a bunion growth.

Along with treatments that are targeted to bunion sufferers, it's a good idea to incorporate additional therapies that encourage overall foot health and comfort.

*Acupressure*   To treat pain in the big toe with acupressure, utilize the Lv3 point, located on the top of the foot in the valley between the big toe and the second toe. Hold the point for one minute, using your thumb or palm.

*Arch support*   Available from shoe repair shops, an arch support is placed in the bottom of the shoe to relieve pressure on the bunion.

*Aromatherapy*   A fragrant and pleasurable way to soothe tired, aching feet is through aromatherapy. Just add ten drops each of juniper and lavender essential oils to two quarts of warm water, then soak your feet for about ten minutes. The soak will not only make your feet feel better, but it can also have the effect of speeding up the healing of mild bunions that are in the acute stage.

*Aspirin wrap*   To remove hard calluses that form on the bottom of the foot in conjunction with bunions, use an aspirin wrap. Crush five or six aspirin tablets into a powder, then add half a teaspoon each of lemon juice and water. Apply this paste to all of the hard-skin areas. Then, wrap your entire foot with a warm towel and cover with a plastic bag. Sit still for at least ten minutes, then remove the coverings and file the callus with a pumice stone.

***Barefoot walking*** A walk on the beach in bare feet can help to get rid of the calluses on the bottom of the foot.

***Massage therapy*** A technique that can help to remove calluses on the bottom of the foot utilizes a mixture of one teaspoon of lemon juice, one teaspoon of dried chamomile tea and one garlic clove that has been crushed. Rub this mixture directly on the callus at least once a day until you obtain results.

***Homeopathy*** The burning sensation in feet, especially around the bunion that is exposed to additional pressure through walking, running or just standing, can be relieved through homeopathic treatment. Commonly recommended is a 6 c dose of apis three times a day. If burning feet feel worse at night, try a 6 c dose of sulphur three times a day. Also, when the burning sensation worsens when walking, try a 6 c dose of graphite three times a day.

Homeopathic substances can also be injected as a way of helping to correct a bunion by irritating the ligaments surrounding the joint so that they will grow stronger and firmer. Substances used include ruta graveolens for sore achy stiffness, strontium carbonicum for joint damage or zeel for tender, damaged joints.

***Lotions and bath oils*** Various lotions and bath oils, especially those with concentrations of lanolin, glycerin or urea, can be smoothed into the feet to soften calluses and roughened skin around the joint. Fruit acid moisturizers are also very effective when heavily applied.

***Massage*** Feet can feel better with massage, especially if they hurt from overuse. Try sitting in a comfortable chair with your left foot crossed over your right leg. Spread a light film of massage oil or vegetable oil on your fingers. Then, with the tip of your thumb, glide along the middle of your sole from the back of the heel to the base of your toes. Repeat this on the right and left sides of your sole. Then, retrace the three lines—middle, right and left—by pressing with the tip of your thumb until the base of your toes is reached. Gently rub and squeeze your toes with your fingertips, paying special attention to the tips of your toes. Repeat with the other foot.

***Stretched shoes***    If your shoes do not allow your feet enough room, they can be stretched. The end of your longest toe should be a finger-width short of the end of your shoe. The shoe itself should be wide enough to allow you to fit a finger between the inside of the shoe and the side of your foot. In front, the shoe should not rub against your big toe or smallest toe. Shoe repair stores have equipment that will stretch any shoes you have that don't meet these standards.

***Nutrition therapy***    The role of nutrition in lessening the effects of bunions has been widely recognized. Of particular importance in overcoming acute inflammation is an enzyme that is combined with several antioxidants called Inflazyme Forte. Although routinely used as a digestive aid, Inflazyme Forte can be a powerful aid in reducing acute inflammation. Suggested dosage is two tablets between meals.

Another valuable nutritional aid in the treatment of a bunion is a combination of calcium and magnesium, in a daily dosage of 1,500 mg of calcium and 750 mg of magnesium, which together help to build and strengthen bones.

Additionally, vitamin C, which promotes the growth and repair of cells, should be taken in large doses during the healing period—some take as high as a total of 3,000 to 8,000 mg daily.

Vitamin A reduces inflammation and aids in the repair of tissues. During the acute phase and for perhaps a month, 100,000 IU daily, then reduce the dosage to 50,000 IU daily and after two more weeks, down to 25,000 IU daily.

Vitamin E also works to reduce inflammation and encourage healing, starting with a dosage of 400 IU daily, increasing to 1,000 IU over time.

## Combined Treatments

Traditional methods for treating bunions have long included many imaginative and practical approaches that are usually more closely associated with alternative methods. One explanation is that surgical treatment is particularly unpopular since a patient's mobility can be greatly affected. Doctors and podiatrists both tend to emphasize a preference for helping a patient prevent escalation of a bunion into a chronic deformity instead of surgery.

Since the bunion is a highly visible ailment, it is fairly simple for a patient to evaluate quickly those therapies that work effectively, including those treatments that are aimed at reducing pain and discomfort.

## Table 8

## TREATMENTS FOR BUNION

| Traditional | Alternative |
| --- | --- |
| **Footwear** | **Acupressure**<br>Lv3 point |
| **Orthotics**<br>mass-produced; custom-fit | **Arch support** |
| **Surgery**<br>open technique; closed<br>technique | **Aromatherapy**<br>juniper, lavender oils |
| | **Aspirin wrap** |
| | **Barefoot walking** |
| | **Food therapy** |
| | **Heating pad** |
| | **Homeopathy**<br>apis; sulphur; graphite; ruta<br>graveolens; zeel;<br>strontium carbonicum |
| | **Lotions and bath oils** |
| | **Massage** |
| | **Stretched shoes** |
| | **Nutrition therapy** |
| | **Pads**<br>sling pad; moleskin pad;<br>separation pad |

# CHAPTER 11

# Carpal Tunnel Syndrome

Carpal tunnel syndrome is a repetitive motion injury whose name reflects the eight bones, known as carpals, that are located in the wrist. The carpals, together with a ligament, form a tunnel-like structure that serves as a passageway for tendons that control finger movement. The tunnel also provides a pathway for the median nerve, which transmits sensations and controls some movements of the thumb and several fingers. Carpal tunnel syndrome is the painful condition that occurs when the tendons become swollen and then compress the median nerve.

Swelling of the tendons can be brought on by the repetitive and forceful movements of the wrist that occur during certain kinds of work and leisure activities. Usually these are activities that involve repetitive manual acts or a prolonged bending of the wrist.

House painters, postal clerks, truck drivers, bank tellers and violinists have been stricken for years. So have carpenters, garment workers, dental hygienists, meat cutters and assembly-line workers. Until only a few years ago, the existence of cumulative trauma disorders was relatively unknown to the general public. In recent years, however, the computer revolution has thrust carpal tunnel syndrome into the spotlight by claiming thousands of new victims and prompting a growing public awareness of its dangers.

Computer operators, of course, are engaged in a highly repetitive activity. The most highly experienced keyboarders are able to type more than thirteen thousand strokes in an hour. Worst of all, these operators often sit in awkward positions and work at keyboards that are too high or screens that are too low. They also may have poor posture or a tendency to strike the keys too hard.

There are many other occupations where carpal tunnel syndrome can occur but it is also especially prevalent within the manufacturing industry in jobs that involve cutting, small-parts assembly, finishing, sewing and cleaning. In all of these jobs, small hand tools are used extensively.

Away from the workplace, activities such as drawing, using power tools, crocheting, needlepoint, gardening, driving, knitting and even wringing clothes can lead eventually to carpal tunnel syndrome.

In addition, the median nerve can be compressed by a ganglion or cyst on a tendon, a tumor or an inflammatory condition such as rheumatoid arthritis. The onset of carpal tunnel syndrome can also be associated with diabetes, an underactive thyroid or a rare disease of the pituitary gland called acromegaly.

It's also possible to contract carpal tunnel syndrome through the accumulation of fluid within certain tissues during pregnancy, from taking birth control pills or by sleeping on your hands or in a position in which the wrists are bent.

Typically, though, carpal tunnel syndrome is the result of daily activities that have kept a person's wrists in a bent position for long periods of time. In the past ten years, the number of cases reported have more than tripled. One reason for this is the degree of automation and job specialization that has taken place, fragmenting workers' tasks so that a given job may consist of only a few maneuvers that are performed thousands of times during a workday.

For example, a worker on a typical assembly-line assembler may perform upwards of twenty-five thousand repetitions a day. When that worker performs the very same motions over and over without any intermittent rest or recovery periods, the damage to the muscles, ligaments and tendons is great.

In addition to the harm that can be caused by prolonged repetitions, workers also need to be concerned about the degree of force or pounding used in their tasks, the unnatural or awkward positions that are undertaken, the force of vibrations at work and the strength of a grip required to hold a tool. Computer operators who pound the keys with abandon, floor polishers who must grip handles very tightly to counteract vibrations, house painters who continually twist and reach in awkward positions; all have elevated risks of contracting carpal tunnel syndrome.

While hands and wrists are the most specific areas in which symptoms of carpal tunnel syndrome are experienced, repetitive strain injury affects the entire upper extremity including the hand, wrist, forearm, upper arm, upper back, neck and shoulder. In such cases, the pain associated with a repetitive strain injury tends to move around from day to day. This migration is made likely because of the body's unconscious ability to compensate for discomfort in one region by having another region take on added work. So, one day you may feel numbness or tingling in one or both hands, and the next day there could be pain in the shoulder or neck.

Not every person will have the same symptoms, while the appearance of one particular symptom may not necessarily mean that the problem is carpal tunnel syndrome. However, if you have several of the symptoms and are engaged regularly in an activity that requires prolonged repetition, strenuous gripping or awkward positions, the possibility should be checked out.

Most common of the early symptoms is a numbness or tingling in one or both hands. Frequently a person will awaken during the night with numbness, tingling or pain. Later on, there may be loss of sensation in the nerves, which will lead to a lack of hand coordination and an inability to hold onto objects. There can also be a problem in performing simple tasks such as tying shoes, turning doorknobs or opening jars, because the hands will seem to lack the necessary strength. Experiencing cold hands regularly, having difficulty just opening and closing them, being unable to differentiate hot from cold by touch and having hypersensitive hands are some other symptoms of carpal tunnel syndrome.

The most dominant symptom of carpel tunnel syndrome is pain. It can be confined to a small place or diffused over a wide area. It can occur when you're just sitting still or it can awaken you during the night. Pain, especially of a chronic nature, should not be ignored.

If you do have symptoms that indicate you might have carpal tunnel syndrome, don't delay seeking out a diagnosis. Getting treatment early on can mean a complete recovery with no lasting effects, while ignoring the symptoms too long could possibly lead to a permanent impairment of your hands.

A doctor will most likely perform a general physical examination of the hand, wrists, forearm, shoulder, back and neck to see if there is swelling, muscle atrophy or tenderness in the muscles and joints. The presence of double-jointedness may be checked out, since it is a frequent characteristic of those who have carpal tunnel syndrome.

There are two tests that are routinely utilized in making a diagnosis of carpal tunnel syndrome: Phalen's maneuver and Tinel's sign. In the Phalen's maneuver test, you place the backs of your hands together, with the tips of the fingers facing the floor and the wrists flexed. Holding this position for about one minute will prompt symptoms of the disorder, if you have it. Using Tinel's sign, also a simple test, you place one hand palm side up and the doctor taps on the wrist at the place where the median nerve is located to see if numbness or tingling occurs.

If the Phalen's and Tinel's results prove positive, an electrodiagnostic test, which studies motor and nerve conduction, is usually performed in order to confirm the diagnosis. A nerve conduction velocity test, it measures nerve damage by passing a low voltage of electricity through certain areas; a damaged nerve transmits the signal at a slower speed than an undamaged nerve. Nerve conduction velocity tests can be uncomfortable but are considered to be very reliable.

## Traditional Treatments

In the 1950s surgery was the only recognized course of treatment for carpal tunnel syndrome. It was a serious and complicated procedure, with an incision made from the palm and continuing all the way to the end of the fingertips. This surgery was followed by a recovery that could take many months. Fortunately, today there are many alternatives available.

Once your physician has been able to evaluate just how serious your condition is, various possible treatments can be considered. An immediate first step is to discontinue immediately those activities that aggravate the symptoms. In reviewing treatment options, the most prudent philosophy is to first consider the most conservative, least invasive procedures. Then, if necessary, begin looking at the more progressively complicated treatments.

*Waiting*   Carpal tunnel syndrome will go away by itself in some cases, usually when the disorder has not progressed beyond early, mild symptoms. All that is required is simply not doing anything other than to completely refrain from any injurious activities.

*Splinting*   When relatively minor symptoms of carpal tunnel syndrome are present, splinting can be an effective method of treatment. Sometimes splints are worn only at night, with the hand and wrist splinted in a neutral position or at a maximum extension of fifteen degrees. In other instances, the splint may be worn at all times. After approximately two or three weeks of wearing a splint, the patient's condition can be reevaluated.

Do rely on your doctor or physical therapist to fit and prescribe the usage of a splint. It is not a good idea to buy a splint from a mail-order catalog or drugstore without medical supervision. Using splints improperly can cause symptoms of carpal tunnel syndrome to migrate. There have also been instances where patients have worn splints and continued to type, which has resulted in the atrophy of some muscles and the overuse of others.

*Medications*   The use of nonsteroidal anti-inflammatory drugs (NSAIDs) can decrease the inflammation and pain and allow the damaged tissue to heal. Use of NSAIDs such as fenoprofen or ibuprofen, along with rest and splinting, can result in complete and full recovery. However, especially for patients over forty, there can be serious side effects from the overuse of NSAIDs, including fever, nausea, ulcers, bleeding, chills, headache, kidney problems and stomach cramps.

The use or cortisone steroid injections, which travel directly into the carpel tunnel often produces dramatic results, with significant reductions in the pain and inflammation of carpal tunnel syndrome in fewer than forty-eight hours. There are serious drawbacks and concerns with this treatment, though, and many physicians strongly oppose the use of steroid injections. Its success depends on extreme accuracy in locating the damaged area. If the injection misses the target, there is little or no result at all; however, if there are repeated injections into the same tendon, there is the possibility of rupturing the tendon.

*Aspirin*   The painful symptoms of carpal tunnel syndrome can be relieved with aspirin, although it should not be used with an NSAID. There are side effects associated with aspirin, which can interact with other drugs, so be sure to discuss its suitability with your doctor.

*Acetaminophens*   Tylenol and other acetaminophens are aspirin substitutes for pain relief that generally do not cause the side effects that aspirins do. Again, check with your doctor before including them in your treatment plan.

*Surgical treatment*   When the condition has progressed to an advanced state and there is a danger of continued nerve damage, surgery is most often recommended. In cases where the pain is relentless and severe and where the thumb has begun to atrophy, surgery is nearly always indicated. Although the surgery is relatively simple and carries little risk of serious complications, it's always wise to get a second opinion from a qualified hand surgeon before deciding to have the procedure.

The objective of surgery is to create more room in the carpal tunnel and thereby release pressure on the median nerve. This is accomplished by dividing the transverse carpal ligament so that it no longer compresses the median nerve as it passes between the ligament and the carpal bones. In some advanced cases, where the lining of the nerve has thickened, it is also necessary to remove scar tissue from the nerve and the lining.

Open carpal tunnel surgery is the traditional method that has been used for nearly fifty years. An incision of approximately two inches is made through the skin covering the carpal ligament, which is then severed. Healing time is about four to six weeks. In recent years, an alternative method using fiber optic tools has been very successful. This "closed," or endoscopic, method involves a smaller incision that is made across the forearm near the base of the hand. Recovery time for this method is about half that of the traditional approach.

There is a new technique, similar to the balloon angioplasty used to open clogged arteries, that has recently been employed in treating carpal tunnel syndrome. A small incision is made at the base of the palm, under the ligament. When the balloon is inflated, it stretches the ligament rather than cutting it and creates additional room for the nerve.

**Physical therapy**   Once the condition has been arrested and the damaged tissue is healing, physical therapy can be beneficial. A physical therapist will utilize deep tissue massage to break down scar tissue, which binds together muscles that ordinarily would operate independently; massage also separates the scar tissue from muscle tissue. Other techniques that are used in physical therapy are heat treatments, stretching, ultrasound and vibrating massage to achieve flexibility in the muscles and tendons.

## Alternative Treatments

Some of the alternative treatments for carpal tunnel syndrome that are widely utilized concentrate on reducing the pain associated with the symptoms. Other therapies focus on the prevention of new or additional symptoms.

*Acupuncture*  The utilization of acupuncture treatments will increase the production of endorphins, the natural painkillers produced by the body, and relieve the painful symptoms of carpal tunnel syndrome. Such treatments also promote a beneficial effect on the healing of the median nerve.

*Vitamins*  A carpal tunnel syndrome patient can benefit from a vitamin regimen in several ways. During the recovery period following surgery, vitamin C can help in the healing process, while vitamin E has been found to minimize soreness and inflammation. However, the vitamin that has created quite a stir as an agent of treatment for carpal tunnel syndrome is vitamin B. Specifically, $B_6$ in a dosage of 300 mg daily for three months has been found to be highly beneficial. It is believed that $B_6$ works to strengthen the sheath that surrounds the tendon and so relieves the pain. $B_6$ treatment is even more effective when it is combined with $B_2$, $B_{12}$ and folic acid. Recommended dosage is 100 mg daily of $B_2$, 1,000 mcg of $B_{12}$ and 800 mcg of folic acid. After three months, you should reduce the B$_6$ dosage to between 50 and 100 mg daily as a maintenance level. It is important to not take more than the recommended amount, because B$_6$ can be toxic at high levels.

***Acupressure*** An effective method of easing the pain of carpal tunnel syndrome is acupressure. Before beginning the procedure, be sure that you are sitting comfortably and have located points P7 on the inside of each arm in the middle of the wrist and TW4 on the outside of the arm in the hollow at the center of the wrist. You can work on the two points at the same time, by placing your left thumb on the TW4 point of the right wrist and the left fingers on the P7 point of your right wrist. Press those points for a few minutes and then switch sides. This procedure can be repeated several times during the day.

A shiatsu form of acupressure, which involves rhythmic pressing for short periods of three to ten seconds, is also effective in countering painful symptoms of carpal tunnel syndrome. In this method, all the fingers are placed on the outside of the forearm, with the thumb on the inside. Begin at a spot about three inches upward from where the crease in the wrist is located. Press on both sides of the bone structure for about ten seconds, then release. Then, move thumb and fingers about a half inch up the arm and repeat. Continue to do this at half-inch intervals up the arm to the elbow. This treatment can be done on both arms several times a day.

***The Alexander Technique*** Many people who suffer from carpal tunnel syndrome can benefit from the Alexander Technique, which develops an awareness of how stress has stifled and inhibited natural body movement. This technique has helped patients to unlearn poor posture habits and to relearn their natural, innate posture, developing a new aware-ness of the head, neck and entire body, and learning bal-anced alignment and automatic movement.

*The Feldenkrais Method*   Practitioners of the Feldenkrais Method believe that the body is able to extend its range of motion and increase overall flexibility and coordination by relearning and reprogramming basic movements. The tech-nique centers around the belief that the skeletal and muscu-lar structures of the body can be trained to move with a minimum of energy and tension, in more natural and health-ful ways of balance and movement. As a result, there will be improved technique at the keyboard for computer users, re-ducing the amount of uneven pressure utilized in striking the keyboard.

*Homeopathy*   The painful joints that are associated with carpal tunnel syndrome, particularly joints that are hot and swollen, may be relieved through homeopathy. Often pre-scribed by homeopaths are bryonia and also rhus toxicoden-dron. For achy muscles, cimicifuga is recommended.

*Progressive relaxation*   Tension in the hand and wrist can be eased by utilizing a technique of progressive relaxation that is quite simple. Begin by clenching one fist as tightly as possible and hold it that way for about ten seconds before re-leasing it instantly and completely. Next, do the same thing with the other fist. Finally, repeat the procedure clenching both fists at the same time. It is recommended that this tech-nique be undertaken before beginning work and then after every break.

*Hydrotherapy*   During the most acute phase of carpal tun-nel syndrome, hydrotherapy can provide much relief, partic-ularly with the utilization of a contrasting bath of hot and cold that improves circulation and reduces swelling. One method is to fill two basins, one with hot water and the other with cold water. First soak your hand and forearm for one minute in the cold water, then soak it for three minutes in the warm. Repeat several times, ending with a cold bath.

*Myofascial technique*   A very specific procedure for treating carpal tunnel syndrome, the myofascial technique involves a combination of stretch and direct pressure. By stretching out the ligaments and tendons surrounding the carpal tunnel, this method is effective in treating mild to moderate cases of carpal tunnel syndrome. However, the technique is not recommended for severe cases. In the procedure, a practitioner first holds the patient's arm out in front with the palm facing up and pulls the thumb back towards the body. Then, the thumb is used as a lever, being pulled and at the same time extended down towards the floor; this process tugs on the ligament and stretches it out.

## Combined Treatments

In coping with carpal tunnel syndrome, you need to concentrate on several phases of treatment. First, there is the immediate need to repair the damage and rehabilitate the injured area. The severity of the damage will greatly influence the choice of which treatment to utilize. It is important to discuss every aspect of the various stages of treatments with your doctor, who can advise you how best to combine traditional and alternative therapies.

Once the injury is stabilized, various treatments can be utilized to strengthen the ligaments and muscles. Finally, the cycle of injury and healing must be broken by concentrating on ways to prevent new injury. You will probably need to retrain yourself and learn new methods of performing those activities that originally provoked carpal tunnel syndrome.

Prevention programs include examining and redesigning tools and equipment; retraining body posture and positions to eliminate awkward stances that are damaging; building in regular breaks from doing repetitive tasks; learning and regularly doing special exercises for stretching and strengthening.

## Table 9

### CARPAL TUNNEL SYNDROME

| Traditional | Alternative |
|---|---|
| *Waiting* | *Acupuncture* |
| *Splinting* | *Vitamins*<br>B, C, E |
| *Medication*<br>nonsteroidal anti-inflammatory drugs (NSAIDS) fenoprofen, ibuprofen; cortisone (steroid) injections; aspirin; acetaminophens | *Acupressure*<br><br>*Alexander Technique*<br><br>*Feldenkrais Method*<br><br>*Homeopathy*<br>bryonia; rhus toxicodendron; cimicifuga |
| *Surgical treatment*<br>open carpal tunnel surgery; endoscopic; balloon angioplasty | *Progressive relaxation*<br><br>*Hydrotherapy*<br>contrast bath of hot, cold |
| *Physical therapy*<br>deep tissue massage, heat treatments, stretching, ultrasound, and vibrating massage | *Myofascial technique* |

# Appendix: Resources and Organizations

Alternative Medical Association
7909 Southeast Stark Street
Portland, OR 97215
(503) 253-4031

American Chiropractic Association
1701 Clarendon Boulevard
Arlington, VA 22209
(703) 276-8800

American College of Sports Medicine
P.O. Box 1440
Indianapolis, IN 46206
(317) 637-9200

American Holistic Medical Association
2727 Fairview Avenue East, Suite B
Seattle, WA 98102
(206) 322-6842

American Massage Therapy Association
1130 West North Shore Avenue
Chicago, IL 60626
(312) 761-2682

American Podiatric Medical Association
9312 Old Georgetown Road
Bethesda, MD 20814
(301) 571-9200

Ankylosing Spondylitis Association
P.O. Box 5872
Sherman Oaks, CA 91413
(800) 777-8189

Arthritis Foundation
1314 Spring Street, NW
Atlanta, GA 30309
(800) 283-7800

Association for Repetitive Motion Syndromes
P.O. Box 514
Santa Rosa, CA 95402
(570) 237-7400

International Institute of Reflexology
P.O. Box 12462
St. Petersburg, FL 33733
(813) 343-4811

Lyme Disease Foundation
P.O. Box 462
Tolland, CT 06084
(800) 886-LYME

National Center for Homeopathy
801 North Fairfax Street, Suite 306
Alexandria, VA 22314
(703) 548-7790

# Glossary

*Acetaminophen* A substance that can reduce the pain and fever of an illness but is not able to relieve swelling.

*Acupressure* An oriental treatment combining aspects of acupuncture and massage techniques, utilizing finger and thumb pressure instead of needles to stimulate certain points on the body to bring about relief for various ailments. The amount of pressure is somewhere between pleasure and pain.

*Acupuncture* A traditional Chinese medical (TCM) treatment that treats disease and lessens pain through the insertion of thin, disposable stainless steel needles into certain points which, when properly stimulated, affect the flow of life energy and the function of related organs, resulting in a restored state of balance.

*Alexander Technique* A method of sitting, standing and walking reclaims the innate posture that has been lost. Focusing on eliminating tension and overcoming bad postural habits, this technique can benefit people who suffer from back and neck pain, spinal disk bulges, pinched nerves and arthritis.

*Allopathic* A traditional practice of medical treatment that is based on evidence obtained through scientific experimentation. Accepted medical procedures must show that a treatment or drug has a measurable, beneficial effect before being utilized by practitioners.

*Alternative medicine* Health methods that are outside the realm of traditional allopathic medicine, including natural or holistic medicine and any therapeutic approach that is not part of the Western scientific medical establishment, the latter being grounded in the traditional disciplines of physics and chemistry.

*Ankylosing Spondylitis (AS)*  A type of inflammatory arthritis which primarily affects the spine and sacroiliac joints and which may lead to progressive fusion of the spine, resulting in loss of spinal mobility. It tends to affect mostly young men and is strongly associated with a genetic predisposition.

*Arthritis*  A word that literally means inflamed joint but is used to identify a group of more than one hundred rheumatic diseases that affect not only the joints but also other connective tissue of the body such as muscles, tendons, ligaments and the protective coverings of internal organs.

*Aspirin*  Acetylsalicylic acid, a substance used to reduce fever, relieve headaches, soothe aches and pains and even ward off strokes and heart attacks. Can irritate stomach if taken too often.

*Ayurveda*  An ancient system of healing based on five thousand years of folk wisdom from India, whereby the human body is a moving stream of submolecular particles that can be arranged and rearranged at will.

*Biofeedback*  A technique in which a person learns through mental concentration to consciously control many normally automatic body functions, such as heart rate, brain rhythms, body temperature and muscle tension.

*Bunion*  A deviation of the big toe, which can cause the misaligned joint to become swollen and tender. The deformity causes the first joint of the big toe to slant outward and the second joint to angle toward the other toes.

*Bursitis*  A disorder that causes inflammation or irritation in the bursae, which are the small sacs—located between bones and muscles, skin or tendons—that promote smooth movement between these structures. This is a common condition, usually temporary but sometimes recurrent, that is often accompanied by severe pain and immobility. Frequent locations for bursitis include the shoulder, hip, elbow and knee.

*Carpal Tunnel Syndrome* A condition that is caused by compression of the median nerve at the wrist, producing pain or numbness in the hand or forearm. It occurs most frequently in people who work at jobs requiring repetitive hand-wrist movement.

*Chi* The life energy that flows through the body along a series of pathways called meridians, according to classical oriental theory, and which is the basis of acupuncture and acupressure.

*Chiropractic* A method of treatment that is based on the belief that health and disease are related to the proper functioning of the nervous system. Therapy involves physical manipulation and adjustment of the spinal column, joints and soft tissues and does not include surgery or medication.

*Electrotherapy* The use of electricity as a healing treatment, by means of electrical muscle stimulation; commonly used to treat muscle strains, sprains and spasms.

*Gout* A form of intense inflammatory arthritis that is caused by deposits of small sodium urate crystals in or around a joint. Gout usually occurs in one or a few joints, with typically the big toe being involved.

*Herbal therapy* A treatment approach that is based on the use of plants that contain healing properties to detoxify the body and rid it of an attacking illness. Plant medicine is also used in the pursuit of overall wellness and to rebuild the body's natural defenses.

*Homeopathy* A healing therapy that is based on the principle that a body's natural defenses can be stimulated by
giving a patient an extremely diluted solution of a substance that normally would bring on the symptoms of the
disease if given to healthy people.

*Hypnotherapy* A technique utilizing the power of hypnosis
on the unconscious mind in order to achieve beneficial
results, such as the mitigation of pain and the lessening of
fear.

*Ibuprofen* A nonsteroidal anti-inflammatory drug (NSAID)
that can reduce fever, relieve pain and soothe headaches
without in most cases also irritating the stomach.

*Inflammation* A localized response to an injury of the tissue, marked by redness, heat, painful swelling and often
a loss of function.

*Joint* Composed of cartilage, joint space, fibrous capsule,
synovium and ligaments. Fixed joints hold the bones together, as in the skull. Partly movable joints allow some
flexibility, as in the spine. Freely moving joints provide
variable flexibility, as in the jaw, shoulder and knee.

*Ligaments* Bands of cordlike tissue that connect bones to
each other.

*Lyme Disease* An infectious illness caused by a bacteria
that is transmitted to humans by the bite of a small tick.
Symptoms include rash, fever, headache, stiff neck,
arthritis, heart problems and neurologic abnormalities.
While appropriate antibiotics can effectively treat the disease, an accurate diagnosis is often difficult.

*Macrobiotics* A combination of diet, philosophy and
lifestyle that originated in Japan and is based on there
being a central life force that puts all living things into
balance. It claims to be able to prevent and treat a num-

ber of diseases, including cancer, heart disease and diabetes.

*Massage* A healing therapy more than five thousand years old, with numerous variations, including deep-tissue massage, neuromuscular massage, tapping, and kneading, light brushing and sports massages. Used to improve circulation, loosen muscles, enhance skin condition, calm the nervous system, relieve chronic pain, increase joint mobility and aid digestion.

*Naturopathy* A healing philosophy that stresses the ability of the body to heal itself, if given the right tools, including rest, vitamins, nutrition, homeopathic remedies, acupuncture, herbal medicine and hydropathy.

*Nonsteroidal Anti-inflammatory Drugs (NSAIDs)* A group of drugs that includes aspirin and aspirinlike drugs; used to reduce inflammation that have caused joint pain, stiffness and swelling.

*Nutritional supplements* Vitamins, minerals, herbs, amino acids and enzymes contained in capsule or tablet form, which are thought to counteract toxic molecules and protect the body against diseases such as cancer and heart disease, as well as help attain maximum health.

*Occupational therapy* A health specialty focused on improving a person's ability to perform daily tasks, facilitating successful adaptation to disruptions in lifestyle and preventing loss of function.

*Osteoarthritis* The most common form of chronic arthritis, affecting more than 16 million Americans, in which the cartilage within the joints deteriorates and results in bone spurs. Symptoms of the disease, which rarely occurs before age forty, include joint pain, loss of function, decreased joint motion and deformity.

*Osteopath* A medical practitioner similar to traditional physician in training and licensing; emphasizes manipulative therapy and drugless techniques but utilizes orthodox procedures as well as surgery, drugs and the latest medical technology.

*Osteotomy* A surgical procedure where bones are cut and repositioned in order to treat diseased or deformed joints or the bones themselves.

*Reflexology* A healing therapy based on the belief that certain spots on the feet are directly linked to other body parts, including muscles, bones and organs; and that massaging these spots can help the body relax and return to a natural balance of good health.

*Rheumatoid Arthritis* The most common form of chronic inflammatory arthritis, characterized by pain and swelling in many joints, affecting more than 2 million Americans. Symptoms include morning stiffness, afternoon fatigue and occasional low-grade fevers. The disease, which is most common in middle-aged women, can cause severe joint deformity and disability.

*Rheumatologist* An internist or pediatrician who is qualified by additional training and experience in the diagnosis and the treatment of various forms of arthritis and other disabling and sometimes fatal disorders of the joints, muscles and bones.

*Support group* A group of people—for instance, cancer survivors, AIDS patients or recovering substance abusers—who share a common condition and develop a bond of trust that enables them to help each other by exchanging advice and offering comfort.

*Systemic* A disease or condition that affects many parts of the body.

*Temporomandibular Joint Disorder (TMD)* A group of painful ailments that affect the jaw joint, muscles and the entire facial area.

*Tendon* A fibrous cord that connects muscle to bone, such as those that move the fingers, thumbs and toes.

*Therapeutic touch* A healing therapy that is based on the belief that a life energy is present in every cell, creating a bioelectric field just above the surface of the body. Practitioners use the hands to sense weaknesses or congestion in the bioelectric field and to restore balance to the body's energy.

*Ultrasound* High-frequency sound waves that are absorbed and reflected at various degrees by tissues in the body. Ultrasound is used for both diagnosis and treatment.

*Yoga* A form of body conditioning derived from an Indian tradition four thousand years old that emphasizes stretches and poses and seeks to unite mind, body and breath. It is thought to reduce mental fatigue, increase rational thinking processes, improve breathing and metabolism, as well as reduce tension and promote muscle relaxation.

# Index

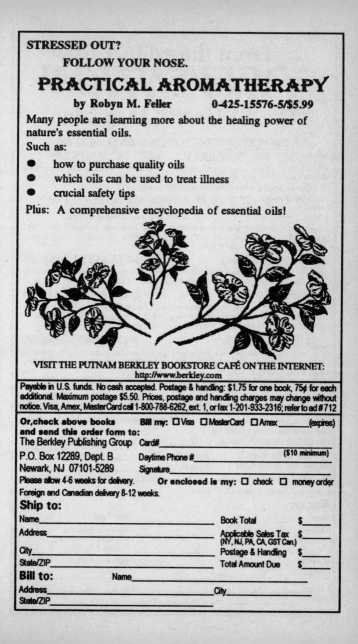